KETOGENIC DIET FOR BEGINNERS

The Complete Guide To Keto Diet
For Beginners Including 7 day Program and
171 Healthy Keto Recipes

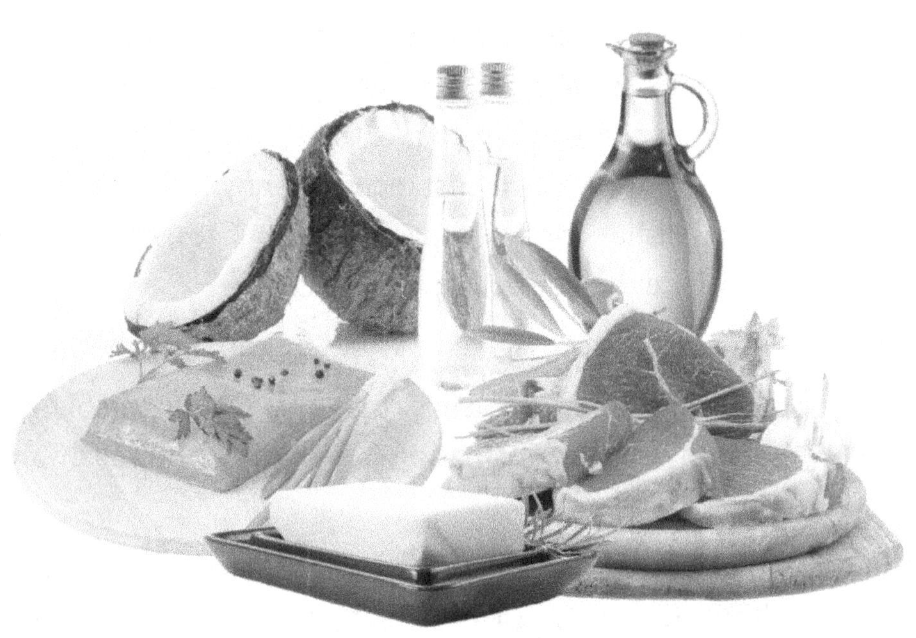

Anna Lovette

Table of Contents

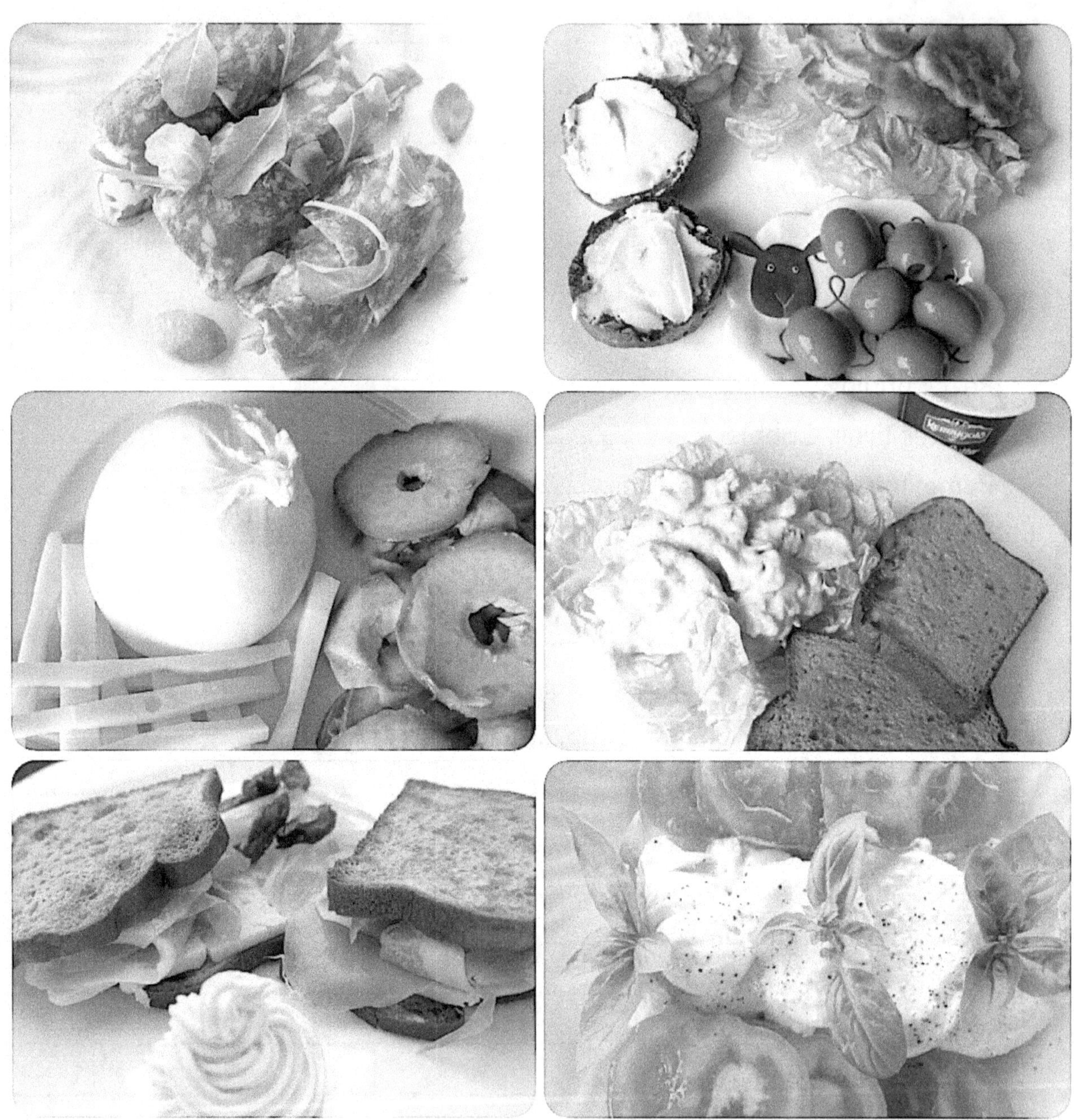

Introduction

Much has been made of all sorts of quick-weight loss, and fad diets, all delivering the promise of a slimmer figure, glowing good looks, and good health forever and ever. Unfortunately, that is all that they deliver: PROMISES. The slimmer figure and good looks may last for a little while, but the good health facet may not even be achieved even if the weight loss objectives are met.

The problem with these diets is that they were only designed for short-term weight loss, and if we really want to talk about diets, we know that over 97% of dieters get back the pounds that they have lost, and in many cases, actually gain more than what they originally weighed in the first place!

That is for only one diet - people spend a lot of their time going on diets, and the results are hardly successful. In a 2007 study, it was learned that women spend, on the average, 31 years of their lives going on a diet; just exceeding the number of years that men spend, 28.

Another problem with diets is that they usually require a drastic change in the eating patterns. Many require a dramatic drop in caloric intake. Some diets require that people eat tasteless and unappealing foods, making them want to end their diets quickly, and they just revert to their old eating patterns.

The diet that I will lead you through, Ketogenic Diet, is not a fad diet, and its underlying principles have been around for decades. In fact, Ketogenic Diet has not only been a sure-fire approach to weight loss. It has been used to treat certain health conditions, and help others avoid various illnesses.

Carbohydrates Explain

<u>Mankind's original fuel</u>

All engines need fuel and energy, and human beings, as the most complicated naturally-occurring engine in existence, is no exception. While we put gasoline as fuel in cars, as human beings, we also need to have our own fuel, and this fuel is food. More precisely, food that will be needed in relatively large amounts, consumed consistently and regularly.

Our fuel, food, is comprised of three basic macronutrients: carbohydrates, fat and protein. Everything we eat as fuel for storage and energy comes from these three macronutrients.   The human body needs these to function properly. How has the consumption of macronutrients changed over the last 10,000 years or so and what has brought us to this world of dieting and more correctly, failures in dieting?

<u>Gog</u>

Let me introduce you to "Gog," a typical ancestor from our prehistoric days, from about 10,000 years ago, give or take a few hundred years. Gog was a male member of the most advanced and latest version of Homo sapiens, of which we eventually became the proud descendants. In that stage of human history, Gog was part of that group called the "hunter-gatherers," who sourced their food from animals that they hunted and killed, and from fruits or berries that they happened to come across in their hunting adventures.

Gog and other co-inhabitants of the planet at that time subsisted on a diet that consisted mostly of animal fats, protein, and fibrous berries and fruits. Their Vitamin D source was principally the sun, and they had little use for plant carbohydrates, from whose chlorophyll content merely transfers the sun's Vitamin D nutrients.

Gog stayed out in the sun for most of the day, and the sun provided his "D". Vitamin D was, and continues to be important to sustain the human's bodily functions, but it is clear that fat was to be the human's primary source of fuel.

It is important to note that even today; certain tribes and cultures subsist on essentially high-fat diets and thrive with robust health. The Maasai group in Africa and Eskimos are modern day cultures that are known for the very small part that carbohydrates play in their diet. These groups are sustained by high fat diets in particularly unforgiving weather conditions. Apparently, their low-carbohydrate lifestyles have turned their metabolisms around to fat burners, rather than glucose burners.

This low-carbohydrate situation seemed to be the way that nature designed humans and their fuel needs: Man got their energy from fat, and fat was their fuel. For millions of years, the genius of nature, or even the genius of a Creator deemed that fat would be man's primary source of energy.

Was this simple diet enough for Gog's sustenance and health? For this, we can look at the archaeological record. On the next page, we present a table that shows life expectancy from the year 9,000 B.C., when agriculture, tilling the soil for carbohydrate foods, is generally is known to have started.

TABLE 1.
Life Expectancy of Our "Lithic Ancestors"

Period of Time	Ave. height-male	Ave. height-female	Life expectancy-Male	Life expectancy-Female
30,000 to 9,000 B.C. (Meat and fat is about 2/3 of the diet)	177.1 (5'9.7)	166.5 (5'5.6)	35.4	30.0
9,000 to 7,000 B.C. (Some agriculture already started – Meat and fat is now less than 1/3 of the diet)	172.5 (5'7.9)	159.7 (5'2.9)	33.5	31.3
7,000 to 5,000 B.C. (Agriculture spreads widely in the Early Neolithic age – Meat is now 30% of the diet)	169.6 (5'6.8)	155.5 (5'1.2)	33.6	29.8
5,000 to 3,000 B.C. ("Late Neolithic," i.e., the transition towards full blown agriculture is mostly complete)	161.3 (5'3.5)	154.3 (5'0.7)	33.1	29.2
3,000 to 2,000 B.C. (Early Bronze Era)	166.3 (5'5.4)	152.9 (5'0.2)	33.6	29.4

The above table shows that when humanity began the agricultural stage, life expectancy actually decreased! The decrease should actually have been bigger if we factor in the increased physical security that our ancestors had because of agriculture: enclosed communities and better defensive mechanisms and positions against predatory animals. In fact, deaths from predators on the general population would be reduced to almost zero, with fatalities coming from predators only occurring with the armed male hordes that elected to hunt for animals.

Gog consumed just what his body required, and most of what he consumed was fat from whatever animals he hunted down. The fat he consumed was burned immediately and quickly, not because of physical activity per se, but because the human body, unlike a car, consumes and uses up energy even while he is in a state of rest and even sleep.

From Chapter 2, we will learn that the carbohydrates he consumed were immediately expended for quick bursts of energy. Gog therefore used his nutrients efficiently and effectively, not requiring much fat to be manufactured or stored. This is something we will come back to later in Chapter 4, when we talk about the mechanics of the diet.

<u>"Post" Gog</u>

The archaeological record also shows that as agriculture began to produce more food, agricultural plant products began to play a bigger role in the human diet. When human beings retreated into safer and cozier settlements, there was less of a need to go out and secure animal foods for food. Also note from the table, that males had higher life expectancies than females, even when their lives appeared to be in more mortal danger, being the hunters.

Humans, especially the male hunters, often turned into prey for the animals of the day. Despite this, males still had higher life expectancies because they presumably ate more of the fat that they hunted, possible consuming much of their meat immediately after securing them, and even before distributing them to their waiting families.

In a couple of thousand years more, meat, and especially fat, would continue to take a backseat to processed carbohydrates. Agriculture would become more efficient, and humans would not only produce more of carbohydrate foods, especially in the form of wheat and rice, they could store these foods longer!

For example, wheat and rice could be pounded down to flour, and stored in silos and bins over long periods of time. Because they could be stored longer, they became a much cheaper and more available source of sustenance and nutrition. After all, why risk lives hunting for food when it could be retrieved in a matter of minutes from a storage bin?

<u>Health problems increase</u>

As time marched on, life expectancies would increase as humankind learned more about medicines, while infant mortality rates would plummet. By the Middle Ages, average life expectancies would approach 50 years or so, but other mortal problems would surface: obesity, heart disease, and metabolic issues. Increased carbohydrate intake would totally throw human metabolic processes into crisis.

Before we get into the science and chemistry of food, we can historically trace these problems to one thing: Humans stopped eating naturally, and more importantly, reduced their intake of fat. Millions of years of eating unprocessed foods and fat were in the millennial blink of an eye, overturned, and the human body was shocked, and not pleasantly, to the new nutritional realities.   Natural and fat was out, processed and carbohydrates were in. So-called blood diseases, and all sorts of unidentified diseases, presumably cancer and diabetes, began to spread.

<u>Modern Man Doubles Down on the Carbohydrate Problem</u>

From the middle ages to well into the 20th century, humankind saw an increasing, if not alarming incidence of heart disease and symptoms reflecting diabetes. Archaeologists, who have studied heart disease not surprisingly, found that heart disease was extremely rare in pre-industrial societies. After the so-called "Industrial Revolution," which gave witness to large-scale mechanization, heart and metabolic diseases shot up, and people were all of a sudden getting sick in newer ways. Heart attacks and symptoms attributable to strokes suddenly took hold.

Modern conventional wisdom, however, attributed this rise in diseases to the sedentary lifestyle that the advances in technology, especially the invention of machines, brought. The thinking was people were getting fatter and sicker, not because of food, but because people were doing less manual labor than from thousands of years ago.   "Experts" assumed that fat deposits formed because people didn't exercise or were sitting, or lying around more.

What they missed or ignored was how human diet was drastically transformed when agriculture took over the human food supply. Modern technology not only made people move around less, it also helped mass produce agricultural products at a faster and cheaper pace.

After wheat and rice were produced in huge, mass proportions, sugar production finally became widespread in the 1700's, and made food, especially, carbohydrates, taste much better. Well into the 1900's, foods high in processed carbohydrate content, such as pizza, French fries, candies, and processed dairy foods gained shot up in popularity.

Moreover, processed carbohydrates became popular because of the short amount of time required to prepare, and with the advent of the microwave oven, cook them. Fast food became a symbol of modern society, and these foods are mostly all about carbohydrates in most of its forms: popcorn, potato chips, and candy bars being the most widespread and popular.

The growth of carbohydrates was largely ignored as a cause of increased heart disease. Because the true villain for human health was being overlooked, a boogeyman had to be found or invented – dietary fat.

<u>Fat gets a bad rap</u>

Sometime in the 1990s, fat was beginning to get demonized. It quickly became the dirty word of the nutrition industry and it was fashionable to shun as a deadly health hazard. Doctors derided it as a scourge to physical well-being, and consumers followed the medical herd, making fat as the primary source of a bunch of physical ailments, most of them revolving around the heart. High "bad" cholesterol, weight gain, artery disease, you name it– all of these were blamed on fat.

The curious thing about the demonization of fat was that there wasn't (and there still isn't) adequate scientific proof to back up these claims of nutritional Armageddon arising from fat.

Despite what science failed to prove, everyone jumped on the low-fat bandwagon, consuming mass quantities of food that, while indeed lacking fat, were instead, loaded with carbohydrates, especially sugar. The results of this "diet revolution" were that the average American got more obese, and the rate of increase of heart problems hastened.

According to U.S. Department of Health and Human Services statistics, by 2001, roughly a third of the American population was already overweight. This, of course, came with the increase in the incidence of heart disease and diabetes also soared.

The result of this "conventional wisdom" was that fresh whole foods such as meat, eggs, and their fatty components—the foods our ancestors ate for centuries—were being quickly replaced with low-fat "Franken foods" such as margarine, low-fat snack cookies, and skim milk. These foods were not only full of sugar and carbohydrates; some were also loaded with artificial ingredients. When these substances are consumed regularly, over time, the human body reacts by gaining weight, showing symptoms of fatigue and brain fog, and succumbing to chronic conditions.

Although scientific research produced findings to the contrary, fat—especially saturated fat—had developed a lasting reputation for being bad. Although the low-fat diet craze eventually dwindled, the damage was done. Fat was shunned and carbohydrates were placed on the nutritional pedestal.

In fact, government authorities began to promote, and still promote, the consumption of mostly carbohydrates, for their recommended dietary combinations. The National Institutes of Health, for example, continue to suggest that 70% of a diet should be comprised of carbohydrates in various forms. Subsequently, in the "Dietary Guidelines for America, 2015-2020," issued by the U.S. Department of Agriculture, dietary fats are merely mentioned almost as a footnote as oils.

The USDA also says that food oils (not fat) are limited to fat in liquid form, while naming vegetable cooking oils as the only source of fat nutrients that should be available for human consumption. There is no mention of the animal fat that our ancestors like Gog consumed, which was actually the main source of his energy fuel. The USDA caps their dismissal of fat by allowing very limited consumption levels of animal fat for the "ideal" diet.

To disseminate this fat-starved diet, the USDA pictorialized their concept of an ideal diet with the "My Plate" diagram, which portrays this dismissal of animal fat from the daily diet. The "Plate" emphasizes vegetables, fruits, grains, and protein, and assigns dairy as a supplemental item on the plate diagram. This diagram suggests that at least sixty percent of a person's recommended calorie intake should be comprised of foods from carbohydrates, which make up grains, vegetables, and fruits.

Fats from non-aquatic animals as beef, pork, and lamb, have been excluded in the nutritional conversation, with the "Plate" admonishing everyone to shun the so-called "trans-fat". Government agencies' objective is to limit the consumption of red meat, cheese, and processed meats.

The USDA recommended "Plate" is depicted as follows:

Source: U.S. Department of Agriculture

Nevertheless, many current scientific studies have not only repudiated the omission of animal fats from the diet, but have argued that fat from animals is not just a necessary component of the human diet, but should be accepted as the largest part of human nutrition. This is especially true when someone is endeavoring to lose weight, and eventually, get healthier.

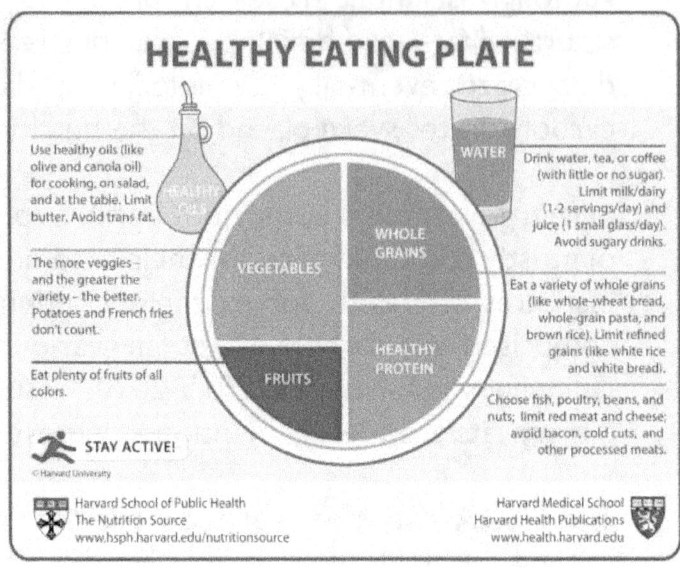

The USDA, the National Institutes of Health, the World Health Organization, our grandparents, physicians, and even our gym instructors have been telling us what to eat. Now after we have followed their recommendations, and of course, our own palate, we consume the food and enjoy them. Sometimes, we don't really enjoy these, but just follow the herd to appear to stay modern and in touch. Regardless of what we eat, certain things happen in our body to convert all those goodies into energy.

We mentioned that food is the fuel that provides human beings with energy. The three macronutrients, carbohydrates, protein, and of course, fat are the fuels that power our bodies 24/7, day in and day out, whether we are moving around, resting, or even sleeping. In this chapter, we see the role of the macronutrients in the sustenance of our bodies, and how food is converted into fuel and other substances in our body.

Our bodies are highly intelligent, and yet, "needy" machines. They know exactly what they want, and more importantly, what they need. The most unconscious of these needs, and yet probably the most important, is the need for fuel to provide our bodies with energy. Without these energy sources, our cells would starve to death.

You see all these shows and movies about people stranded in islands, forests, and deserts without food? Those are the consequences when you're conscious minds and bodies cannot get the fuel necessary to function, and endure.

The first step, the easy and conscious part; chewing and swallowing, puts food into our bodies. The next, more important, however subconscious step; happens inside our body -- to break down this food for absorption, and conversion into energy. This process is called metabolism.

<u>Eating up</u>

Metabolism describes the chemical reactions that take place to maintain the dynamic state of our bodies and their constituent cells. Metabolism has two subordinate bodily functions to process the food/fuel, which we can conveniently divide into the following:

Catabolism– This refers to the breakdown of the molecules that we ingest. The macronutrients are broken down in substances and molecules that can be usable for the body to convert into fuel and energy.

Anabolism - This refers to the amalgamation of all compounds needed by the human body. Basically, in this stage, the body takes what has been broken down by catabolism, and processes the molecules to convert them to energy.

When we ingest the foods that contain the macronutrients of carbohydrates, fat, and proteins, our bodies immediately begin to work on the foods that we take in. The last conscious effort we have in this process is the swallowing of the foods that we have either chewed or drunk. When the mass of chewed food and/or liquids have passed our throat, and heads down our esophagus, the rest of body takes over beyond our conscious control. What happens to these foods?

In order to make sure that it always has access to energy; our body has several metabolic pathways it can use to convert the food that we eat into useable energy, and energy that we can store. We will summarize what these metabolic pathways are all about in the rest of this chapter.

For human beings, the default metabolic pathway is one that uses the glucose from carbohydrates as fuel. As long as you provide your body with carbohydrates, it will use them as energy, and storing excess macronutrients as fat in the process. When you deny your body of carbohydrates, it has to turn somewhere else to get the energy it needs to live. For millions of years up to about 9,000 years ago, the human body turned to mostly, stored and dietary fat.

<u>Anabolism– fed and fasting states</u>

In the metabolic process, a distinction also has to be made between the "fed" and the "fasting" state when the nutrients are being broken down during the anabolic stage. The fed state occurs about 4 hours after eating a meal or snack.   This is the time when the body begins to absorb the digested nutrients. Some of these nutrients, especially carbohydrate-based ones, are used to meet immediate energy needs, while converting the extra nutrients to energy stored products.

In the "fasting state," which occurs 4 or more hours after eating, the body uses fat as its main source of energy. How fat or thin we are, depends on how much of fat stores are used, and of course, how those stores are built.

Let us now discuss these blessed little fuel sources.

<u>Carbohydrates</u>

These are probably the tastiest of all foods, the "lightest" on the mouth and the palate, the easiest to swallow, and from an economic standpoint, the cheapest. Rice and wheat for example, can be expanded to 2 or 3 times their original uncooked mass, then laced and mixed with all manner of sugars, creams, flavors, and texturized ingredients to provide the tastiest satisfaction from the lips to the tongue.

After we ingest carbohydrates, these are immediately broken down, by the introduction of various enzymes, into glucose, which is basically blood sugar. Some of the glucose is burned for instant energy, but usually, there is excess glucose left in the blood stream to trigger the body to try to regulate these increases in glucose.

Glucose is the body's favorite source of energy on demand, and is the fuel of choice for athletes, bodybuilders, and gym rats. This is why we have "sugar boosts" after consuming an energy bar or cookie, after a workout or an athletic exercise. The metabolic process that glucose undergoes is called "glycolysis," where the glucose is converted to mostly glycogen.

In the human body's infinite wisdom, it knows that too much glucose can be a problem (which we will see in a while.) To regulate the level of blood sugar, the body lets the pancreas release insulin, a regulating hormone. From this we can see that nature has considered carbohydrates to be inherently bad for the human body, otherwise, why limit it?

Indeed, nature has planted an organ in our body, the pancreas, to produce a singular hormone, insulin, to prevent the body from taking on too much blood sugar. We will visit insulin again in the next chapter when we talk about the effects of sugar and fat on the body.

<u>Proteins</u>

Proteins are responsible for creating the "building blocks" of our body tissues. The most common forms are lean meats and certain legumes. The foods containing protein provide more of a "chewing" sensation before being swallowed, provide the most "filling" sensation, and are more expensive per ounce, than carbohydrates.

Proteins are broken down into amino acids, and used by body cells to form either new proteins or to mixed up in some kind of amino acid "pool". This pool serves like a cache for the molecules, creating some sort of reservoir. Amino acids comprise a significant percentage of our body mass. A big percentage of our cells, tissues, and muscles are also comprised of amino acids.

Amino acids, therefore, perform a bunch of key body functions. One of the most paramount is giving our cells their form and structure. The metabolic process that protein undergoes is called "transamination," where the amino acids we eat are converted to glycogen or other protein compounds.

Aside from forming body tissues, amino acids play an important part in the storage and transport of essential nutrients. They have significant influence over the functions of arteries, glands, organs, and connective tissues, such as tendons. They also are indispensable for repairing tissues, and healing wounds, most especially in the skin, hair, bones, and muscles. Proteins also play an important role in the elimination of various waste deposits arising from metabolism.

Just as ingesting too much of carbohydrates is an issue, the body will need to "dispose" of "extra" amino acids produced over and above the body's requirements. The excess amino acids are transformed by enzymes in the liver into urea and keto acids. These keto acids can then be utilized as extra sources of energy, and via different anabolic processes, are transformed into glucose, or stored in the muscles as fat.   Urine and sweat takes care of eliminating urea from the body.

<u>Fat</u>

Fat can be yummy, and can be gross at the same time, but fat is the king of human body fuels; nature having decreed it as the best source of energy. Fat from foods usually is ingested as part of other food items. For example, one can eat the fatty part of steaks, the skin of chickens, and the fat from fish, and egg yolks. Pure fat can be taken in limited forms: of such foods as whole milk and fried eggs.

When fats are eaten, they are converted into fatty acids and glycerol. They are digested in the person's small intestine. They are then turned into lipoproteins for different essential functions (we will talk about bad and good cholesterol, LDL and HDL in the next chapter).

<u>Getting energy from carbohydrates, proteins, and fat</u>

When you eat, the nutrient molecules are absorbed in the intestine and into the bloodstream. In the fasting state, the cells will soon be taking up these nutrients and chemically burn them to liberate energy. The most common chemical fuel is the sugar glucose. Other molecules, such as fats or proteins, can also supply energy, but they usually have to first be converted to glucose or some intermediate that can be used in glucose metabolism.

This is where the energy superstar, adenosine triphosphate, or ATP, comes in. After all the three macronutrients are metabolized, ATP, a critical element in human metabolism, is produced when the body burns the sugars together with other nutrients. Mitochondria in the cells convert the food that we eat into ATP, which is a comparatively smaller molecule which functions as "energy intermediate" when we metabolize food.

ATP is often referred to as "chemical currency" as the body uses it as a direct energy source. The body produces ATP when it burns up various nutrients and sugars, while our cells ingest ATP when engaging in actions such as producing movement, and on an atomic scale, building larger molecules. Our cells then chemically process ATP, resulting in the release of energy, in order for the human body to engage in various activities.

In essence, our body cells take out the chemical energy from different nutrient molecules such as proteins and carbohydrates, and then utilize this chemical energy to produce ATP.   How do we go from glucose to ATP? This is achieved through the process of "oxidation".

For example, glucose, the molecule that came from our consumption of carbohydrates, including many dietary sugars and starch, are broken down to make waste products like water and carbon dioxide. But our cells will utilize the energy freed up from breaking down a single glucose molecule, and produce about thirty ATP molecules.

As soon as a cell has produced ATP, it will now utilize the ATP to meet any of its energy requirements. Cells require energy in order to produce large molecules, such as hormones, for example. Muscle cells also make ATP to generate movement. As a cell produces a large molecule, ATP molecules are broken down. The cell utilizes this energy to produce original bonds among smaller molecules resulting in the production of a bigger one, and the process goes on.

All these processes occur amazingly without our conscious effort or thinking.   Our bodies are amazing machines that do all these processes automatically.   If we take in the right foods in the right amounts, there shouldn't be any problems.   However, since the age of agriculture dawned on humanity 9,000 years ago or so, our bodies have unfortunately, not been so lucky.

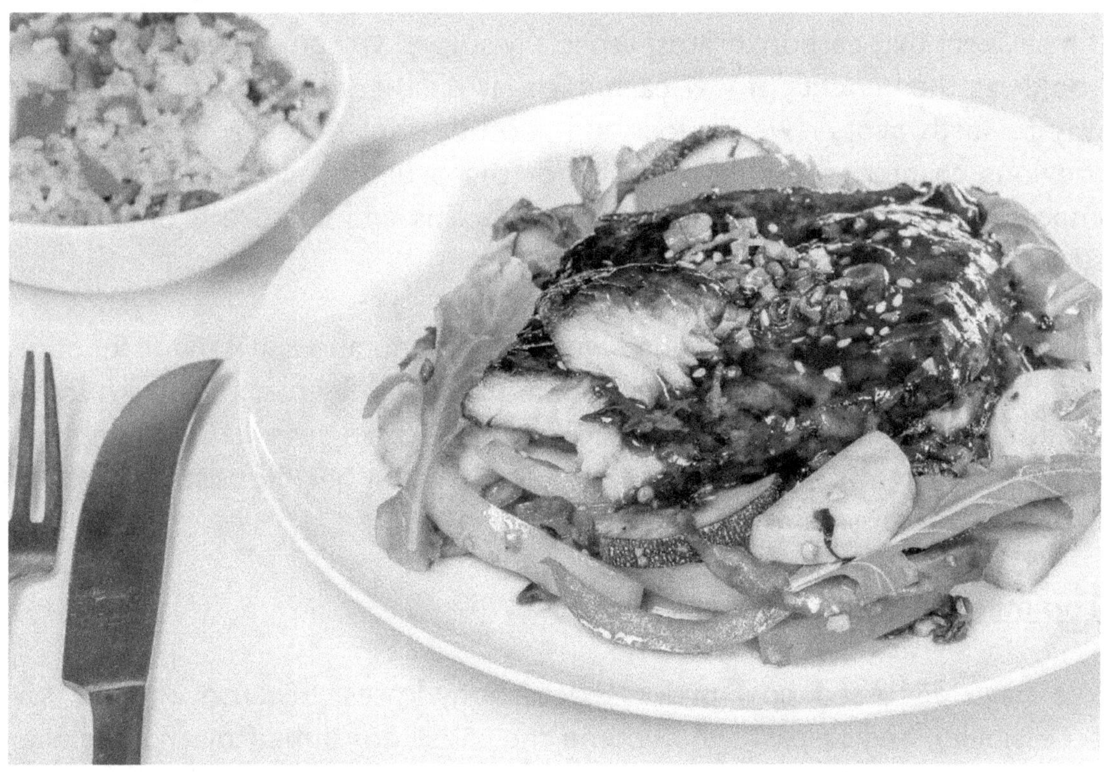

We now have an idea of how the body processes the macronutrients.   Let us pay attention to the negative side of eating, and what happens when we take in too much of the "wrong" types of food into our bodies, especially carbohydrates. In the previous chapter, we mentioned that our bodies were "intelligent" in the singular sense that it tells us when we need fuel, and signals our bodies to take in food whenever our energy sources are getting low.

On the flipside, however, our bodies cannot be "smart enough" to totally withstand bad nutrition, which is eating foods that were not originally designed for our consumption. Despite our bodies' best "efforts," we become obese and sick, and there is very little that it can do from a self-defense standpoint to fight this. In nutrition, the worst thing that can happen to the human body, aside from not being fed enough, is being fed too much, and worse, being fed too much of the wrong foods.

<u>The sugar curse</u>

It may seem that carbohydrates, especially sugars, will be demonized in this, and other books, as the benefits of low-carb, high-fat diets continue to portray as the correct way towards proper weight loss and good health. Actually, as we have seen in the previous chapter, sugar by itself, is not the problem. In fact, we talked about the importance of glucose, and how even proteins and fats are broken down to make sugar in the body.

Glucose is absolutely essential to life, and our metabolism cannot function properly without it. Each cell in our body is able to utilize glucose as energy. Even when we cannot obtain glucose from our diet directly, we can get what we need from fats and proteins. In fact, we have a constant supply of it in our bloodstream. But it can also create severe problems.

<u>Too much sugar</u>

We have discussed how processed carbohydrates, because of their lower price, accessibility, and taste, have become the most consumed macronutrient. The fact that they are also the "lightest" on the mouth and the palate, added to carbohydrates' promotion as the preferred macronutrient, it has practically ensured that human beings will eat them more than any other food.

But sugary and carbohydrate-packed foods are also the most easily converted and metabolized macronutrient. They pass through the digestive tract the fastest, and these factors combined ensure that too much of carbohydrates can be eaten, especially if the habit is picked up when we are young. The bottom line is that anytime we fill our bodies with more than the needed fuel levels, the storage capacity of our liver for sugar is exceeded, and sometimes, greatly.

The liver can store up to only around 5% of its mass as glycogen, which has been converted from excess glucose. When the liver is packed at close to full capacity, the excess sugars are transformed by the liver into more fatty acids.

Worse, these fatty acids go back into the bloodstream, and is distributed throughout our bodies and stored as fat! These fats are stored away where our bodies are designed to store these as adipose fat cells. These areas include, but not limited to, the popular regions of the butt, breasts and hips for women, and the stomach for men. These fatty cells can also imbed themselves in the arteries, causing arteries to deteriorate and being clogged with fat and debris from extra fat.

As a disastrous reverse bonus, as soon as these areas become full with fatty tissues and adipose cells, they will start to leak over into our vital organs– these include the kidneys, liver, and heart. The presence of fat will impair and impede the organ's ability to perform, raise blood pressure, lower metabolic rates, cause a feeling of constant tiredness, and expose the body to illness and sickness as our immune system is weakened.

The body pushes excess glucose into the cells to be made into ATP, or stored as glycogen which are converted into fat droplets called triglycerides in the fat cells, or adipose tissue. "New fat" has just been created.

<u>The wrong sugars</u>

Compounding the "too much" sugar problem is that we may not only be eating too much of carbohydrates, but humans, more than ever, are consuming the wrong carbohydrates. "Gog" and our prehistoric ancestors filled their bellies with natural berries, natural wild fruit, and natural fibers. The operative was natural, and Gog only ate foods that nature provided.

Today, however, there are a vast multitude of foods that contain sugars that nature did not intend us to ingest. Many foods, especially desserts, have sugar (sucrose) and high fructose corn syrup. These are sweetening agents that help enhance the taste of many foods and drinks— practically all non-diet sodas and ice creams contain them.

These are very different from natural sugars that contain glucose, which is an essential life giving nutrient, taken in the right quantities, but fructose is another matter. The molecule is not part of our normal metabolism and we do not produce it. A tiny fraction of cells in the human body can make use of it except liver cells. Since these cannot be properly assimilated into other cellular functions, they get turned to fat, and are eventually secreted into the blood.

<u>Insulin and the Big D- Diabetes</u>

We mentioned in the previous chapter that our bodies are intelligent enough to know that carbohydrates, and especially, processed sugars, are not good for the body, and it takes great pains to try to mitigate the effects of bad dietary habits. One of its best defense mechanisms is the pancreas, which secretes insulin to help mitigate the creation of too much blood sugars and fats, the results of which can be devastating, as we have seen above.

Insulin plays an indispensable role in the body. Its biggest role is its interaction with glucose to let our bodies utilize glucose properly as energy. The pancreas, the organ which produces insulin, excretes enough insulin and it acts as some sort of a "key" that allows the cells of the body to take in, and use glucose as energy.

Insulin assists in controlling blood glucose levels by alerting muscle cells, fat cells, and the liver to extract glucose from the blood. If our bodies have sufficient energy, insulin alerts our liver to process the incoming glucose, and store it as glycogen.

The glucose that insulin "pushes" in to the cells in the form of glycogen can then be transformed into ATP, or stored as fat as described earlier. This additional stored glycogen can then be utilized later on when the body needs more energy. When our bodies experience a disruption in the balance between fat production and the secretion of insulin, diabetes will occur.

<u>Type1 Diabetes</u>

This form of diabetes has also been called insulin-dependent diabetes or juvenile-onset diabetes, and accounts for less than 10 percent of all diabetes cases. Usually a genetic affliction, in this diabetes type, our body's immune system kills the cells that are responsible for releasing insulin, which in effect, stops insulin production.

<u>Type 2 Diabetes</u>
This is the type that Ketogenic Diet will most likely try to address. Type 2 diabetes is the most common form of diabetes (over 90% of diabetes cases), and is usually the result of a diet with very high in carbohydrates. The ones suffering the disease will manifest any symptom prior to diagnosis. Usually Type 2 diabetes is found during adulthood, although a few cases have been known to have been diagnosed in children.

In this affliction, our bodies cannot process insulin the right way. While the most common root cause is still debatable, there is a growing consensus that this is a "lifestyle" disease emanating from an overconsumption of carbohydrates. The bottom line is that the ability of the body to produce insulin has been overwhelmed by the amount of glucose produced. This condition is called, "insulin resistance," and eventually, the body will make less and less insulin, leading some to require insulin injections.

Since Type 2 Diabetes is a lifestyle disease, the way to deal with it is to change our lifestyles! This is best done by going on Ketogenic Diet, and getting the body into the ketosis state.

Ketosis And Ketogenesis

The human body was designed to use fat for energy, and when mostly fat is used for energy, it does not store that fat, and the body becomes lean, as nature designed it. From Chapter 2, we found out that our bodies have several metabolic pathways it can use to convert the food that we eat into useable energy. The default metabolic pathway is one that uses the glucose from carbohydrates as fuel. As long as you provide your body with carbohydrates, it will use them as energy, storing fat in the process.

When you deny your body with carbohydrates, it has to turn somewhere else to get the energy it needs to live. If you starve your body of carbohydrates, therefore, the body will burn fat, and in the metabolic process, it will produce something called, "ketones." These are what may save your life!

Ketones are organic compounds that are made in the liver from fatty acids, and are generated from the breakdown of fats, especially when the body cannot "locate" any glucose to turn into energy. Ketones are formed almost as a defensive action by the body. When it "senses" that there is not enough sugar or glucose to provide for the body's energy needs, it immediately creates an alternative fuel source.

<u>The Creation of Ketones and Ketosis</u>

During times of fasting, or when we intentionally follow a low-carbohydrate diet, it turns to fat for energy.   In simple terms, fat is taken to the liver where it is broken down into glycerol and fatty acids through a process called beta-oxidation. The fatty acid molecules are further broken down through a process called cytogenesis, and a specific ketone body called acetoacetate is formed.

If we continue on Ketogenic Diet, over time, our bodies will adapt to using ketones as fuel, and our muscles will convert the acetoacetate into beta-hydroxybutyrate or BHB. BHB is actually the preferred ketogenic source of energy for your brain, and acetone, most of which is expelled from the body as waste.

When dietary carbohydrates are suddenly taken away from the diet, more fatty acids are released from fat cells, which leads to more fat cells being burned up in our liver.

This increase in the burning of fatty acids in the liver eventually causes ketone bodies to be produced, and induces ketosis, a new metabolic state.

Other hormones are likewise affected, and these help transfer the use of this new fuel, instead of carbohydrates, to body tissues. The majority of calories burned up by the human body will now come from this fat breakdown.

The glycerol created during the beta-oxidation process enters into a stage called gluconeogenesis. During gluconeogenesis, the body converts glycerol into glucose that your body can use for energy. Your body can also convert excess protein into glucose. Your body does need some glucose to function, but it doesn't need carbohydrates to get it. In other words, during this period, our body is beginning to now burn fat instead of converted sugar! Ketosis has set in, and hopefully for good!

<u>So is fat and ketosis bad?</u>
Ketogenic Diet has been at the forefront of a big diet "revolution" for the past few decades. Its popularity continues to increase, as new scientific evidence continues to surface, and proves that fat does not deserve the bad nutritional reputation it has received. Is fat bad?

The human body was designed to use fat for energy, no matter where it is produced. This results in a lean body, as nature originally designed it. How does a dieter on Ketogenic Diet get to ketosis? Getting to a state of ketosis means ingesting less than 50 grams of carbohydrates per day, and in the next Chapters we will find out how to count these carbohydrates, including the tools you need to measure carbohydrate intake.

<u>Weight loss in Ketogenic Diet</u>

Now that you understand how your body creates energy and how ketones are formed, you may be still be wondering just how this translates into weight loss. Let's provide a quick review and summary.

When you eat a lot of carbohydrates, your body happily burns them for energy and stores any excess as glycogen in your liver, or as triglycerides in your fat cells. When we take carbohydrates out of the equation or reduce our intake of them drastically, our body depletes its glycogen stores in the liver and muscles and then turns to fat for energy.

When our bodies start to burn stored fat, our fat cells shrink and you begin to lose weight and become leaner. Smaller, leaner cells = smaller, leaner bodies!

Ketosis has sometimes been confused with ketoacidosis, which is a pre-existing condition present in some diabetic patients. It is a condition where there is not enough insulin produced in the body. Ketosis is not ketoacidosis, and vice-versa. Ketosis will not lead to ketoacidosis, and assuming you have no other medical conditions that may prevent you from going on Ketogenic Diet.

While many people try to dismiss Ketogenic Diet as a dangerous fad diet, it is well worth noting that the diet has many helpful, life-changing, and life-saving effects on our bodies and long-term health. Weight loss and looking great is sometimes viewed as merely side benefits by those who have stayed on the diet for an extended period of time.

There are other ways on how Ketogenic Diet can contribute to your well-being and long life.   If you understand what amazing benefits are in store, it will be very easy to get convinced to stay on the diet. Described below are the foremost benefits of going on Ketogenic Diet.

Elimination of Type-II diabetes

We mentioned that Type-II diabetes is a lifestyle issue, and that it can be cured by a lifestyle change. For diabetes, the best lifestyle change is to get on Ketogenic Diet, and stop letting carbohydrates ruin your health. Many Type-II diabetes conditions are treatable before requiring the use of injected insulin.

Reduction of the symptoms of epilepsy

Ketogenic Diet is sometimes recommended to help control seizure symptoms in some patients afflicted with epilepsy. Ketogenic Diet is prescribed by a doctor and the patient undergoes careful monitoring under the watch of a professional dietitian.

Reduction in the symptoms of cancer

Cancer cells are very much not like our healthy cells. One way that they have known to be way different is that they have about ten times as many more insulin receptors on their surface as ordinary cells. The receptors allow the cells to feed on nutrients and glucose coming from the bloodstream at a very significant rate.

The more carbohydrates that are catabolized, the more glucose are produced which helps the cancer cells gorge for their "nutrition." If we are able to remove carbohydrates from our diets, we can possibly deny cancer cells from their energy source.

<u>Reducing the incidence and severity of Parkinson's disease and Alzheimer's</u>

Parkinson's disease is one of those "motor system" disorders where the onset happens between the ages of 50 and 65 years old. In the United States, about 1 percent of people in that age group are affected with it. In Parkinson's disease, the dopamine-producing cells in the brain are seemingly destroyed. The symptoms of Parkinson's disease include slowness of movement, trouble with balance, tremors, and shaking.

Near the terminal phase, the victim is usually on a wheelchair, or bed-ridden. These symptoms show up after up to 80 percent of the dopamine-producing cells in the brain are devastated. While it is not exactly clear on how Ketogenic Diet can alleviate the symptoms of Parkinson's disease, it is highly possible that ketones, which have an anti-inflammatory effect on the brain, may be able to fix impaired neurons.

The ketones may also possibly bypass the area in the brain that is damaged, and bring much-needed energy to other areas in the brain.

<u>Reduction of symptoms of Mitochondrial Disorders</u>

Mitochondria are organelles that are of significant numbers in most human cells. This is where the essential biochemical processes of energy production and respiration take place. Mitochondria are also considered as the energy centers of the human body. They convert the food that we eat to adenosine triphosphate, or ATP, as we have learned in Chapter 2.

When mitochondria become dysfunctional, the cells are denied of the energy they need. Because the brain, muscles, heart, nervous system, and eyes demand the most energy, their cells are often the most significantly affected with a mitochondrial disorder. Affecting these body parts cause learning and intellectual disabilities, muscle weakness, hearing and visual impairment, respiratory disorders, and even seizures. There is no cure for mitochondrial disorders, so their treatment focuses on alleviating its symptoms and improving the quality of life of the sufferer.

Proper diet is often the first stage of therapy for these disorders, and with seizures are a common symptom, a high-fat, Ketogenic Diet is often part of the treatment plan.

<u>Reduction of symptoms of Lou Gehrig's or ALS Disease</u>

ALS (Amyotrophic Lateral Sclerosis) is a progressive, neuro-degenerative ailment that assaults the nerve cells in the spinal cord and brain. ALS specifically affects the motor neurons, which are responsible for voluntary muscle movement. When motor neurons die, they are no longer able to send nerve signals to the muscle fibers leading to slurred speech, difficulty swallowing, muscle weakness, and almost instantly fatal breathing. At any rate, most of the muscles begin to waste away, and the person affected becomes weaker.

The exact cause of ALS is unknown, and there is no cure for the disease. Researchers believe that disruptions of the mitochondria in the brain and changes in a person's diet may help those with ALS, as well. Studies on mice and other animals show that those under Ketogenic Diet experienced a greater decrease in symptoms than those who weren't.

Improved Focus and Mental Clarity

For the brain, exposure to too much glucose can result in neurotoxicity or the exposure of the nervous system to toxic substances. Many mental issues, such as brain fog and problems with memory, are caused by this condition. In Ketogenic Diet, the reduction of the supply of glucose diminishes the levels of toxicity in the body as brain starts to use ketones as fuel.   Possible results are the ability to think more clearly, better focus, and better memory recall.

Increased Energy

When the body breaks down fat instead of carbohydrates, more energy is produced for each ounce of fat used, leaving the Ketogenic dieter with a feeling of heightened alertness and increased energy.

Better heart and coronary health

When there are less fat cells flowing through the blood stream, that means that there is less strain on the heart and the arteries. This is a result of less plaque clogging up the bloodstream, and a better functioning circulatory system.

Lower "bad cholesterol" levels

Weight and fat loss are the objectives of an overwhelming majority of people going on Ketogenic Diet. Of course, the associated benefits of a slimmer body can also lead to a decrease in "bad" cholesterol levels, blood pressure, and just better heart health.

Breaking the myths surrounding high fat diets

It is useful to know what people, even health professionals, can say to scare people from Ketogenic Diet. There are many myths and misconceptions that have surrounded, and clouded ketosis and Ketogenic Diet.

Ketosis myths

Myth 1: Carbohydrates are an essential nutrient for good health.

Myth2: Eating a low-carbohydrate diet can lead to vitamin deficiencies, especially Vitamin C, which come from carbohydrate-rich sugary fruits and vegetables.

Myth 3: Ketogenic Diet causes your body to go into ketoacidosis, which is dangerous.

Myth 4: Your kidneys will sustain damage from high fat consumption.

Myth 5: A high-fat diet will lead to osteoporosis, because it will cause the body to excrete calcium.

Myth 6: Eating fat makes you fat.

Myth 7: Ketogenic Diet leaves out carbohydrates completely.

Myth 8: Cholesterol from animal fat causes heart diseases.

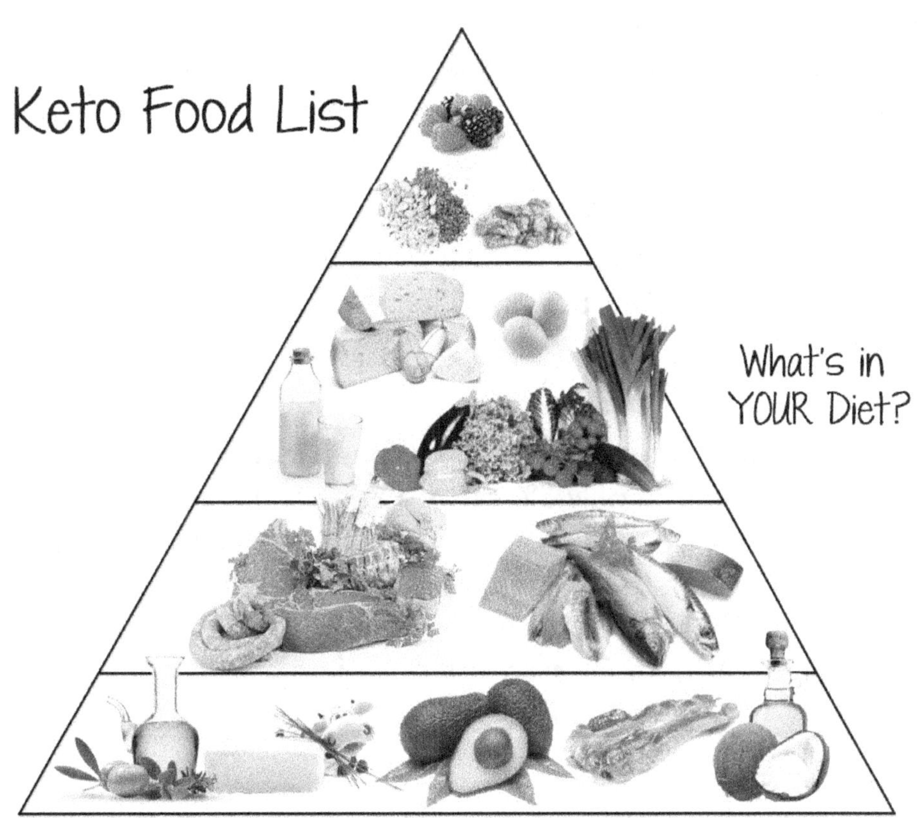

Put quite simply, the Ketogenic diet is a high-fat, low carb, moderate protein diet. Got it? Great. Now let's get into the specifics. It is really quite simple. Once you get started on it, you'll find it to be very intuitive.

All human bodies require three main macronutrients to survive: carbohydrates, proteins, and fats. For years, we have been taught that we need to eat a high carb, moderate protein, and low fat diet. But what has that really lead to? High rates of obesity, sickness, and poor health across the board. Eating high carb leads people to go on binges, eating too much, and making themselves sick. What if we change our thinking, and entirely change the focus of our diets?

The Keto diet changes the focus from carbs to fat. On a Keto diet, you want your intake to be very high-fat, with close to zero carbohydrates. Most Keto practitioners eat 80% of their daily calories from fat. So what does that look like?

1 gram of fat has 9 calories. So if you're operating on a 2,000-calorie diet per day, you need 80% of that to come from fat. 80% of 2,000 calories would be 1,600 calories, or 178 grams of fat per day. Don't worry, there isn't this much math involved in day-to-day Keto eating!

Okay, but what about the other two macronutrients? On a Keto diet, you'll eat 80% fat, 15% protein, and only 5% carbs. Let's continue with our 2,000-calorie example. 1 gram of carbohydrates and protein both have 4 calories. On a 2,000-calorie diet, you'll want 15% to be protein, which works out to 300 calories, or 75 grams of protein. Carbs are even less — 5% of your 2,000 calories. That ends up being only 100 calories, or 25 grams of carbohydrates.

Before we get into the nitty-gritty of the diet, an important few words on how Ketogenic Diet is different from other low-carbohydrate diets on the market.

<u>Atkins Diet</u>

Atkins Diet was at the forefront of the low carbohydrate revolution and brought ketosis and ketogenesis into public awareness about fifty years ago. Atkins Diet allows for a moderate amount of protein in the menu. The allowable ratio is about 50-35-15 in terms of fat/protein/carbohydrate ratio. In Ketogenic Diet, the overwhelming amount of calories should come from fat, about 70%.

Atkins Diet also puts a lot of emphasis on the two week, "induction" phase, where the dieter will have to consume the required macronutrients. Atkins Diet promoters claim that a pers0n can lose up to fifteen pounds on the first week of the diet.

Atkins Diet also allows the dieter to slowly reintroduce certain carbohydrates after the induction period.   On Ketogenic Diet, the dieters need to be on a high fat diet for the rest of their lives.

Paleolithic Diet

Paleolithic Diet focuses on the foods supposedly eaten by our prehistoric ancestors, just like Ketogenic Diet, and also reduces the emphasis on carbohydrates. But Paleolithic Diet also allows for more significant portions of vegetables and certain fruits. Certain grains are allowed, and in fact recommended. Like Ketogenic Diet, Paleolithic Diet forbids tubers and sweet potatoes. The big difference between both diets is that high fat dairy products can be consumed on Ketogenic Diet, but is expressly disallowed on Paleolithic Diet.

Other diets that promote lower carbohydrate intake

Two other famous diets, Zone Diet and South Beach Diet, also recommend carbohydrate intake significantly lower than that of Ketogenic Diet. However, they allow for the consumption of a wider variety of carbohydrates.   Ultimately, only Ketogenic Diet dictates that the significant majority of macronutrients consumed should be from fat.

The importance of macronutrients

Our body's overwhelming source of fuel is the food that we eat. Some of our energy comes from sunlight (Vitamin D), but 99% of our fuel comes from macronutrients in the food that we eat. Ketogenic Diet's effectiveness depends almost wholly on what we eat and drink.   There is no need for supplementation, such as vitamins when we go on Ketogenic Diet.

Think of the macronutrients as the gasoline that we put in our cars. Taking in the wrong macronutrients can be compared with putting contaminated fuel in your gas tank, or putting diesel fuel, for example, in a car that requires high-octane gasoline.

In Ketogenic Diet, the proper fuel is fat.

Getting on Ketogenic Diet

a. Prepare your household and cupboard for Ketogenic Diet

Going on a high-fat diet means a big change in lifestyle. If we are not living alone, and have to share our cupboards, refrigerators, and shopping budgets with other people, we need to properly announce that things will be changing drastically in the food storage department.

On Ketogenic Diet, carbohydrates are the big enemy, and we have to make sure that no "stealth carbs" manage to intrude our food space. Be organized, create lists, and shop carefully. We go into much greater detail on what we need to eat in the next chapter.

<u>b. How many grams of protein, carbs and fats should be eaten in Ketogenic Diet?</u>

We mentioned that most "authorities" recommend that about two thirds of calories should come from carbohydrates. This means that for a typical daily diet of 2,000 calories consumed, at least 1,300 calories of the total should be consumed in the form of carbohydrates.   Additionally, around 500 calories should come from protein, and the remainder, should come from incidental, and trace quantities of fat.

Remember that these so called authorities do not even contemplate fat as being a food group, but only gives some token credit to fats as oils added to foods for taste and use in food preparation.

Ketogenic Diet turns this all around. Dietary fat should now make up about two-thirds of daily calorie consumption, allowing a maximum of ten percent to come from carbohydrates. Converting this to food weights, this means that under Ketogenic Diet, we should only consume daily between 30 and 50 grams of carbohydrates.

The more active a person is, however, a little more carbohydrates are added, maybe up to 100 grams, can be eaten. This is a concession to the fact that carbohydrates are useful for those that require short-term bursts of energy, such as those who go to a gym or exercise regularly and athletes.

For protein, the recommended quantity can be between 115 grams and 175 grams per day. The rest of the diet should be concentrated on fat. For a 2,000 calorie daily diet, we need to ingest at least 60%, or 1,200 calories of fat, 25%, or 500 calories from protein, and 15%, or 300 calories, from carbohydrates.

A note on protein which we have given very little attention to: Proteins are important in the creation, maintenance, and repair of muscle tissues. We want protein to rebuild our tissue, and not be an inefficient source of energy. In fact, excess proteins can turn into fat, the way carbohydrates are converted.

<u>c. Recording and monitoring calorie and macronutrient intake</u>

To ensure of the success of the diet, we need to carefully monitor how much of each macronutrient we are consuming daily, to ensure that the right proportion of calories are being consumed.

There are a multitude of carbohydrate/calorie counters that are available. The preeminent source is the suite of Atkins Diet publications that pioneered the high-fat revolution. These need to be purchased in publication or app form.

Regardless of whether you record your progress in a written journal, or monitor yourself via computer, tablet, or phone, you need to strictly be in compliance with the percentages I have just mentioned. This monitoring is especially important in the first few weeks, when you are transitioning your body into the ketosis state.

Of course, you need to pay strict attention to the actual macronutrients you can (and should not!) consume when you are on the diet.

<u>d. Signs That You Are in Ketosis</u>

Signs that you're in ketosis may start appearing after only one week of following a true Ketogenic Diet. For some people, it can take longer—as much as three months. The amount of time it takes for you to start seeing signs that your body is burning fat for fuel largely depend on you as an individual. When signs do start to show, they are pretty similar across the board.

<u>"Keto Flu"</u>

"Keto flu" or "low-carb flu" commonly affects people in the first few days of starting Ketogenic Diet. Of course, Ketogenic Diet doesn't actually cause the flu, but the phenomenon is given the term because its symptoms closely resemble that of the flu. It would be more accurate to refer to this stage as a carbohydrate withdrawal, because that's really what it is.

When you take carbohydrates away, it causes altered hormonal states and electrolyte imbalances that are responsible for the associated symptoms. The basic symptoms include headache, nausea, upset stomach, sleepiness, fatigue, abdominal cramps, diarrhea, and lack of mental clarity, or what is commonly referred to as "brain fog."

Carbohydrate addiction is a real thing. Some research shows that carbohydrates activate certain stimuli in the brain that can be dependence-forming and cause addiction. Carbohydrate addicts have uncontrollable cravings for carbohydrates, and when they do eat them, they tend to binge. For a carbohydrate addict, the removal of carbohydrates can cause withdrawal symptoms, such as dizziness, irritability, and intense cravings.

The duration of the symptoms varies—it depends on you as an individual, but typically "keto flu" lasts anywhere from a couple of days to a week. In rare cases, it can last up to two weeks. Some of the symptoms of the "keto flu" are associated with dehydration, because in the beginning stages of ketosis you lose a lot of water weight.

With that lost fluid, you also lose electrolytes. You can replenish these electrolytes by drinking enhanced waters (but make sure they are not sweetened) and drinking lots of homemade bone broth. This may help lessen the severity of the symptoms.

<u>Bad Breath</u>

Unfortunately, bad breath is another early sign that you're in ketosis. When you're in ketosis, your body creates acetone as a waste product. Some of this acetone is released in your breath, giving it a fruity or ammonia-like quality. You can combat bad breath by chewing on fresh mint leaves and drinking plenty of water, since bad breath is also associated with dehydration.

<u>Decreased Appetite and Nausea</u>

As your body adapts to Ketogenic Diet, you may have a decreased appetite. This is because you're providing your body with plenty of fat and protein, which are both highly satiating, and not a lot of carbohydrates. The nausea associated with "keto flu" can also decrease your appetite. When you reach this stage, it's important that you eat even if you feel like you aren't hungry. You want to make sure your body is getting enough calories and nutrients, especially in this time of transition.

<u>Increased Energy</u>

When the fog begins to clear and your body starts to become keto-adapted, the uncomfortable symptoms you were feeling will dissipate and you'll begin to see the benefits of following Ketogenic Diet. One of the first beneficial signs many people experience is an increase in energy. When your body breaks down fat instead of carbohydrates, more energy is produced gram for gram, leaving you feeling alert and energized.

<u>Other Possible Signs</u>

Cold hands and feet

Increased urinary frequency

Difficulty sleeping

Metallic taste in the mouth

Dry mouth

Increased thirst

Now let's talk about the cost of the Ketogenic diet. If you're determined to eat all organic, high quality meats and fish of a wide variety, with vegetables bought at specialty markets, and the highest quality nuts and seeds, then yes. It will probably be pretty expensive.

But if you're on a budget, trying to get healthy, and you want to try the Ketogenic diet, I have good news: you definitely still can make it work! There are tricks and tips to making Keto more affordable.

Try buying frozen vegetables and meats, then preparing your meals ahead of time. By buying frozen bulk vegetables instead of fresh, you can have vegetables that stay edible for longer, without compromising on quality or nutrients.

Some meats, also, are cheaper than others. Make the decision to take time at the grocery store and buy the affordable options that are still rich in nutrients. Take the time to find the best deal, comparing the price per pound or gram. It might mean you'll spend an extra 20 minutes in the grocery store, but after a few weeks of this, it'll become second nature.

With frozen vegetables, a few delicious canned sauces (don't forget to read the nutrition label), and a freezer full of fish and meat, you'll be able to eat Keto, lose weight, and save money!

Yep, it's really that simple. Keto is for everyone, so make the right decision and commit to this incredible diet.

Shopping for the right foods is the first and most important step short of putting the right food in the mouth. For today's food shopper, fortunately, most food manufacturers are sensitive to the needs and requirements of people who go on special diets such as Ketogenic Diet. In labeling their foods, they have endeavored to be more accurate and responsive to people who need the proper information to go on their diets.

Regardless of whether foods are "allowed," the serious dieter will still have to make sure that they are staying well within the required macronutrient ratios (preferably 65% fat, 20% protein, and 15% carbohydrates). If measuring ratios are not possible during a given meal, the overriding principle is that the majority of the calories eaten daily should come from fat, and a very small percentage should be from carbohydrates.

<u>Quality</u>

The "quality" of your food matters, especially when it comes to fat and protein sources. Going back to the prehistoric time, our ancestors got healthy on unprocessed and unrefined food alone. It would be healthy and beneficial if a diet plan replicates that prehistoric food profile. A Ketogenic dieter should also try to purchase foods that have the following descriptions on the labels: organic, grass-fed, free-range, and/or pasture-raised.

Food with labels that say, "farm-raised" should be avoided as much as possible, because in all probability, whatever has been "raised" in those "farms" have been sprinkled with a healthy dose of chemicals and preservatives to improve yield and increase the animals' sizes.

Meats, poultry, and seafood

These are the staples of Ketogenic Diet, not vegetables, rice, or grains. They are the most plentiful, and in fact, appetizing components of the diet, and contains naturally-occurring fat. There are many foods in this group that most people can eat all they want every day. Foods included in this food group comprise all types of beef, chicken, turkey, duck, fish, lamb, pork, shrimp, crab, and lobster.

Of course, "exotic" varieties such as ostrich, goat, deer, and buffalo, are also allowed, if available. While bacon and sausage are excellent sources of protein and fat, care should be taken in eating processed meats, especially hotdogs and sausages. Many brands contain substantial quantities of carbohydrate fillers.

Remember that when eating meat, make sure to stay within your recommended protein grams for the day, since your body converts excess protein into glucose via glucogenesis, which can kick you out of the ketosis state.

In the following lists, we will show what the carbohydrate and fat contents are for a particular food item. Remember that these measurements are for uncooked and undressed food. Because Ketogenic Diet is ultimately a low-carbohydrate diet, we are listing the carbohydrate content of each food item. We will also list the number of calories for each item. Note that there may be many varieties of food types, especially in the meat items, because meat comes from various parts of the animal.

The list below is a fairly large general representation of foods that we generally eat. In the reference section of this book, I provide some resources for carbohydrate and calorie counting, in general.

a. <u>Foods that are good for Ketogenic Diet</u>

Animal Meats:

Beef/Veal – 3 oz. has 0 carbohydrates, and about 300 calories

Pork - 3 oz. has 0 carbohydrates, and about 200 calories

Lamb - 3 oz. has 0 carbohydrates, and about 175 calories

Goat - 3 oz. has 0 carbohydrates, and about 100 calories

Venison -3 oz. has 0 carbohydrates, and about 150 calories

Other wild game:

Keep in mind, the organic and grass-fed meat. Even if they are a little more expensive, they are the healthiest options, because there is a much lesser chance that they will contain growth hormones and preservatives. Game meat has generally less calories than regular pork and beef, and for the most part, has zero carbohydrates.

Processed meats:

While being basically comprised of the same meats that we have just listed that have zero carbohydrates, the curing and processing required to give them taste, sometimes necessitates the adding of carbohydrates.

Bacon – 3 oz. has less than 2 grams of carbohydrates, and about 45o calories

Bologna – 12 gram slice has about 1 gram of carbohydrates, and about 50 calories

Pork rinds - 3 oz. has 0 carbohydrates, and about 300 calories

Salami - 12 gram slice has about 1 gram of carbohydrates, and about 50 calories

Sausage (e.g., Bratwurst, Kielbasa, etc.) - 3 oz. has 2 grams of carbohydrates, and about 300 calories

Make sure that these yummy meats do not contain added sugars or excess preservatives.

Poultry:

You can be liberal with the skin and the fat portions. There is no need to skim them off anymore. Once again, organic and grass-fed cuts are the healthiest options. These include:

Chicken – 100 grams has 0 carbohydrates, and about 120 calories

Duck - 100 grams has 0 carbohydrates, and about 130 calories

Goose - 100 grams has 0 carbohydrates, and about 160 calories

Ostrich - 100 grams has 0 carbohydrates, and about 110 calories

Pigeon -100 grams has 0 carbohydrates, and about 200 calories

Quail - 100 grams has 0 carbohydrates, and about 150 calories

Turkey - 100 grams has 0 carbohydrates, and about 125 calories

Speaking of poultry, eggs, especially the yolk part, are highly recommended. Organic eggs or eggs from grass-fed chickens are preferred.

Fish – fatty varieties, especially:

Bass - 100 g has 0 carbohydrates, and about 150 calories

Halibut - 100 g has 0 carbohydrates, and about 110 calories

Mackerel - 100 g has 0 carbohydrates, and about 200 calories

Salmon - 100 g has 0 carbohydrates, and about 140 calories

Tuna - 100 g has 0 carbohydrates, and about 150 calories

Trout - 100 g has 0 carbohydrates, and about 150 calories

Peanut Butter – Check the labels to ensure that the variety is very low in carbohydrates, and have no sugar content. 2 tbsps. Of such varieties have about 5 g of carbohydrates, and 200 calories.

Dairy:

Butter – 0 carbohydrates and 500 calories per 100 grams

Cheese – Make sure that you watch out for blends! They may have sugars and other dangerous chemicals and preservatives to make them look, and taste like real cheese. Most well-prepared cheese without any fillers 100 g has 1.5 g carbs, and about 400 calories

Plant products:

Asparagus, green – 1 cup has 5 g of carbohydrates and calories

Avocados - 1 cup has 20 g of carbohydrates and 300 calories

Bamboo shoots - 1 cup has 8 g of carbohydrates and 40 calories

Broccoli - 1 cup has 6 g of carbohydrates and 30 calories

Celery stalks - 1 cup has 4 g of carbohydrates and 15 calories

Coconuts – 1 cup has 12 g of carbohydrates and 300 calories

Green, leafy vegetables, such as bok choy, lettuce, Swiss card, radicchio, endives. These are non-starchy vegetables and typically 1 cup has about 5-10 g of carbohydrates and between 25-50 calories.

Kale - 1 cup has 5 g of carbohydrates and 30 calories

Kohlrabi - 1 cup has 8 g of carbohydrates and 40 calories

Radish - 1 cup has 2 g of carbohydrates and 15 calories

Broth, especially self-made bone broth, non-sweet pickles, kimchee, sauerkraut, and mustard.

Almost all herbs and spices (no sweeteners and preservatives) and recipe enhancers such as lime juice, lemon, and their grated skins.

Whey protein - keep away from those with sugar, chemical additives, and soy additives

Nuts (make sure there are no sugar-based additives) such as Brazil nuts, hazelnuts, pecans, walnuts, sunflower seeds, sesame and pumpkin seeds, pistachios, pine nuts, and peanuts.

Oils such as coconut oil, pure lard, and olive oil

<u>b. Take the following in moderation</u>

These can be eaten after the initial phase of ketosis has been completed.

Plants:

Bell peppers, shallots, tomatoes - 1 cup has between 10-20 g of carbohydrates and 30-50 calories

Berry varieties, including strawberries, blackberries, cranberries, raspberries, and blueberries. Berries are tricky because while they have an abundance of sugars, they are rich in fiber, which greatly reduces their "net" carbs, or carbohydrates discounted by the fiber they contain.

Cabbage, cauliflower, broccoli, fennel, rutabaga, turnips, Brussels sprouts, and eggplant

Eggplant - 1 cup has 5 g of carbohydrates and 20 calories

Garlic -1 teaspoon has 1 g of carbohydrates and 4 calories

Leeks – The bulbs and lower leaf portions - 1 cup has 15 g of carbohydrates and 50 calories

Mushrooms - 1 cup has 2 g of carbohydrates and 15 calories

Olives - 1 cup has 5 g of carbohydrates and 20 calories

Rhubarb - 1 cup has 5 g of carbohydrates and 20 calories

Onion - 1 cup has 10 g of carbohydrates and 40 calories

Other Peppers- 1 cup has 10 g of carbohydrates and 40 calories

<u>c. Foods that should be avoided at all costs</u>

Alcohol in most forms. Most pure rums and some vodkas though, have zero carbohydrates. Bar beverages and alcohol-based drinks usually have a lot of sugars and syrups and should be avoided.

However, dieters can also consume a variety of beverages in moderation, as long as they contain no sugar. Check the labels carefully on so-called diet sodas to make sure that they do not contain any sugar. Unlimited drinks will include tea, coffee, and heavy cream, minus any refined sugars or sweeteners.

As with most diet plans, water is still the best bet as a beverage alternative. It is a good idea to drink at least half of your body weight in ounces. Plain water can be infused with fresh herbs, such as mint or basil, to provide a little variety. Sodas, flavored waters, sweetened teas, sweetened lemonade, and fruit juices should be avoided.

High-fructose corn-syrup is that deadly stealth sweetener found in most soft drinks, and juices. We mentioned fructose briefly in Chapter 2. If the "high" in high-fructose is not enough to scare someone away, consider that it also functions like a preservative, meaning that not only does it lack B vitamins and other important nutrients, it is chock-full of chemicals that have no business being in the human body.

Avoid grains and sugars in all of their forms. Grains include wheat, barley, rice, rye, sorghum, and anything made from these products. This means that Ketogenic Diet will have no breads, pasta, crackers, and rice. Sugar and anything that contains sugar is also not allowed. This includes white sugar, brown sugar, honey, maple syrup, corn syrup, and brown rice syrup.

There are many names for sugar on the ingredient lists. It's extremely beneficial to familiarize yourself with these names so you will know when a product contains sugar in any form. Be careful of artificial sweeteners like Splenda that could actually be made out of sucralose, which contains carbohydrates.

Breads, including wheat bread

Breakfast cereals

Chocolate bars and candies

Desserts, especially cakes, pies, and pastries

Energy bars, including protein bars

Energy boost drinks - look for sugarless varieties though

Ice cream

Oils that are processed are generally harmful to the body, and will impede Ketogenic progress. These include margarine, sunflower, cottonseed, safflower, canola, grape seed, soybean, and corn oils.

Pancakes and waffles

Rice

Sodas and sugary drinks, including most juice drinks

Syrups and chocolate toppings

T.V. dinners

The basic rule is this: You have to avoid foods and drinks with sugars, carbohydrates, and chemicals.

Tips to Eat More Good Fat

If you try to get all the fat in your diet from fatty meats, you may find that your ratio of fat to protein quickly goes the wrong way. Keep in mind that a high protein diet can lead to glucose in the bloodstream, knocking you out of Ketosis. It's important to supplement your meat intake with other forms of healthy fats.

So, what are some sneaky ways to increase your fat intake? Try piling avocado on top of your dishes. Make oil heavy salad dressings. Cook your vegetables in full-fat butter. Cook your vegetables in a tablespoon of coconut oil. Remember the healthy fats we talked about earlier in the book? Coconut oil, vegetable oils, butter, lard, and healthy plant-based fats like avocado will all help improve your ratio of protein to fat in your diet, and they will also fill you up at mealtime.

MCT Oil

MCT stands for medium chain triglycerides. Sounds complicated? Don't panic. This isn't as horrifyingly scientific as it sounds. MCT Oil is a natural oil found in palm and coconut-based oils. This oil has a remarkable ability to limit glucose and enhance the production of Ketones in the body. If you're looking for oils to cook with, the best one to go with will always be coconut oil, for its amazing ability to make your body produce more Ketones!

Other great ways to include MCT oils in your diet include adding it to salad dressings, mixing it into coffee or tea, or including a tablespoon of oil in your smoothies.

Sleeping during Ketosis

One side effect of Ketosis can oftentimes be insomnia, or the inability to sleep. This happens due to the lack of carbohydrates entering the body. Of course, carbohydrates give us energy, but they also give us dietary sources of tryptophan, a chemical that relaxes us and helps us sleep. Without this, it becomes more difficult to get a good night's rest.

You can offset this Keto insomnia by taking a tryptophan supplement. It may not fix the problem right away, but it should help over time. Other things that can help are increased mindfulness and meditation, as well as high levels of exercise.

While Ketogenic Diet can provide some awesome benefits, there are many pitfalls to avoid if one is to have success, and even avoid serious hazards to your health.

<u>Mistakes on going on Ketogenic Diet</u>

Because Ketogenic Diet is a radical departure from what most people are used to, it is easy to make mistakes. The following are the most common mistakes that can remove the benefits of Ketogenic Diet, and may even cause harm to your body:

1. To gain the maximum benefits from the diet, you have to be in a state of ketosis for at least two weeks. You CANNOT deviate from this, or you will basically need to start from zero again.

2. Eating too much processed fats and proteins. This is especially true for boxed or T.V. dinners. While they may have a lot of fat content, there are usually a lot of hidden sugars, and worse, artificial chemicals that can derail your progress.

3. Eating more protein as opposed to fat. Fat is the main source of energy, and eating excess protein is bad, because some of it is converted to sugar.

4. being afraid of fat. In the dietary world, fat is a friend, and we need to forget all the misconceptions about it.

5. Not getting enough water. Sometimes we drink water to accompany carbs, especially sweets, so drastically reducing carbs may cause us to consume less water. Water is the most important element of any diet, and it sometimes helps to give the body a feeling of "fullness."

Congratulations! You've gone this far, and now it's time to be rewarded for your persistence and attentiveness.

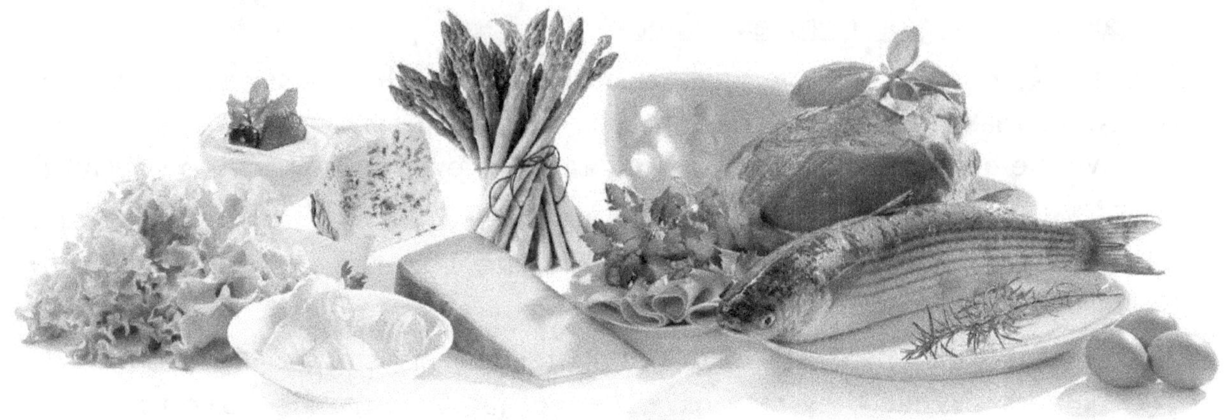

The Advance Ketogenic Diet Recipes
Advance Keto Beef Recipes
Spicy Steamed Meatballs

Serving: 4

Ingredients:

- 1 – pound ground beef
- Half-Cup chopped collard green
- One-teaspoon paprika
- One-teaspoon chili
- Two-tablespoons almond flour
- Two-organic eggs
- 1/4 – teaspoon pepper
- One-teaspoon minced garlic
- Half-Cup low sodium beef broth
- 1/4 – Cup coconut milk

- Two-tablespoons red chili flakes
- Two-tablespoons chopped leek

Instructions:

- Prepare an oven-safe dish and coat with cooking spray.
- Pour beef broth and coconut milk into the dish then seasons with minced garlic and pepper. Set aside.
- Place the ground beef in a food processor together with collard green, paprika, chili, almond flour, and eggs. Process until smooth.
- Shape the mixture into ball forms then arrange them in the prepared dish.
- Pour water into the Instant Pot and place a trivet in it.
- Place the dish on the trivet then covers and seals it properly.
- Select the *Manual* setting then cooks for 20 minutes.
- When the Instant Pot beeps, naturally release it and open the lid.
- Transfer the meatballs to a serving dish together with the gravy.
- Sprinkle chopped leek and red chili flakes.

!

Nutrition Info Per Serving:

- Calories: 296
- Total Fat: 13.7g
- Saturated Fat: 6.6g
- Trans Fat: 0g
- Cholesterol: 183mg
- Sodium: 212mg
- Potassium: 593mg
- Total Carb: 3.2g
- Dietary Fiber: 1g
- Sugars: 1.2g
- Protein: 38.8g

Serving: 4

Ingredients:

- 1 – pound grass-fed beef
- One-teaspoon sliced garlic
- One-teaspoon sliced shallots
- 1/4 – teaspoon pepper
- 1/4 – teaspoon cumin
- Half-teaspoon ginger
- One-inch galangal
- One-bay leaf
- Three-teaspoons smoked paprika
- Two-tablespoons low sodium soy sauce
- Two-tablespoons tomato puree
- One-Cup low sodium beef broth

Instructions:

- Place the beef in an Instant Pot then sprinkle sliced garlic, sliced shallots, pepper, cumin, ginger, and smoked paprika over the beef,
- Add galangal and bay leaf into the Instant Pot then drizzles soy sauce and tomato puree over the beef.
- Pour low sodium beef broth into the pot then cover the pot with its lid. Seal it properly.
- Select the *manual* setting then cooks on high for 30 minutes.
- Once the Instant Pot beeps, quick release the Instant Pot then opens the lid.
- Using two forks, shred the cooked beef into pieces then transfers to a serving dish.

Nutrition Info Per Serving:

- Calories: 284
- Total Fat: 20.6g
- Saturated Fat: 8.1g
- Trans Fat: 0g
- Cholesterol: 80mg
- Sodium: 574mg
- Potassium: 129mg
- Total Carb: 2.8g
- Dietary Fiber: 0.6g
- Sugars: 0.8g
- Protein: 22.1g

Serving: 4

Ingredients:

- Two-pounds beef oxtails
- One-teaspoon pepper
- One-teaspoon nutmeg
- Three-cloves
- Three-cups water
- Half-Cup chopped carrots
- Two-tablespoons chopped leek

Instructions:

- Select the *Sauté* setting of an Instant Pot then pours avocado oil into it.
- Once it is hot, stir in minced garlic then sautés until brown and aromatic. Press the *Cancel* button.
- Add beef ribs into the pot then pours water into it.
- Season with pepper then covers the Instant pot properly.
- Select the *Manual* setting then cooks on high for 30 minutes.
- When the Instant Pot beeps, quick release the Instant Pot then opens the lid.
- Quickly stir in the chopped collard green then mixes until the vegetable is wilted.
- Transfer to a soup bowl then enjoy hot!

Nutrition Info Per Serving:

- Calories: 437
- Total Fat: 23.1g
- Saturated Fat: 9.2g
- Trans Fat: 0g
- Cholesterol: 188mg
- Sodium: 350mg
- Potassium: 77mg
- Total Carb: 3.3g
- Dietary Fiber: 1.2g
- Sugars: 1g
- Protein: 52.8g

Serving: 4

Ingredients:

- 1 – pound beef tongue
- Two-teaspoons minced garlic
- Half-teaspoon ginger
- One-teaspoon pepper
- Two-tablespoons avocado oil
- 1/4 – Cup tomato sauce
- Two-tablespoons diced radish

Instructions:

- Pour water into an Instant Pot then place a trivet in it.
- Combine minced garlic, ginger, pepper, and avocado oil in a bowl then mix until incorporated.
- Peel the beef tongue then rubs it with the spices mixture.
- After that, place the beef tongue on the prepared trivet.
- Cover the Instant Pot with the lid and seal it properly.
- Select the *manual* menu then cook on high for 20 minutes.
- Meanwhile, place tomato sauce and diced radish in a microwave–safe bowl then microwaves on medium until warm. Mix until combined.
- Once the beef tongue is done, quick release the Instant pot then open the lid.
- Transfer the cooked beef tongue to a serving dish then drizzle tomato mixture on top.
- Serve with any kinds of green, as you desired.

Nutrition Info Per Serving:

- Calories: 340
- Total Fat: 26.3g
- Saturated Fat: 9.4g
- Trans Fat: 1g
- Cholesterol: 150mg
- Sodium: 156mg
- Potassium: 305mg
- Total Carb: 2.3g
- Dietary Fiber: 0.8g
- Sugars: 0.8g
- Protein: 22.4g

Serving: 6

Ingredients:

- 1 – pound chopped grass-fed beef

For The Marinate:

- Three-teaspoons lemon juice
- One-teaspoon pepper
- 1/4 – teaspoon ginger

For The Sauce:

- Two-teaspoons minced garlic
- Two-teaspoons sliced shallot
- Three-teaspoons garam masala
- 1/4 – teaspoon paprika
- 1/4 – teaspoon turmeric
- 1/4 – teaspoon cayenne
- One-Cup low sodium beef broth
- One-Cup coconut milk

Instructions:

- Combine lemon juice, pepper, and ginger in a bowl then mix well.
- Rub the beef with the spices mixture then marinates for about an hour. If you have papaya leaves, you can wrap the beef with the papaya leaves. This helps the beef to be tender and juicy.
- After an hour, choose the *sauté* mode on an Instant Pot then stir in the beef. Sauté until the beef is no longer pink.
- Add the remaining spices mixture into the Instant Pot together with minced garlic, sliced shallots, garam masala, paprika, turmeric, and cayenne.
- Pour beef broth over the Instant Pot then covers with the lid and seal it properly.
- Select the *manual* menu then cook on high for 20 minutes.

- Once it is done, quick release the Instant pot then open the lid.
- Select the *sauté* menu again then pour coconut milk over the beef. Stir until the gravy is thickened then transfers to a serving dish.

Nutrition Info Per Serving:

- Calories: 277
- Total Fat: 23.2g
- Saturated Fat: 13.9g
- Trans Fat: 0g
- Cholesterol: 54mg
- Sodium: 190mg
- Potassium: 162mg
- Total Carb: 3.4g
- Dietary Fiber: 1.1g
- Sugars: 1.5g
- Protein: 15.3g

Special Tasty Beef

Serving: 4

Ingredients:

- 1 – pound grass-fed beef
- 1/4 – teaspoon pepper
- 1/4 – Cup avocado oil
- Two-tablespoons Dijon mustard
- Half-teaspoon nutmeg
- One-teaspoon cinnamon
- 1/4 – teaspoon ground cloves

Instructions:

- Cut the beef into thick slices then sprinkles pepper over the beef. Set aside.
- Select the *sauté* setting in an Instant Pot then add the beef in it.
- Brown each side of the beef then presses the cancel button.
- Place Dijon mustard, nutmeg, cinnamon, cloves, and avocado oil in a bowl then mix well.
- Pour the mixture over the beef then covers the Instant Pot and seals it properly.
- Select the *manual* setting then cooks on high for 30 minutes.
- Once it is done, quick release the Instant Pot then opens the lid.

- Transfer to a serving dish then serves immediately.

Nutrition Info Per Serving:

- Calories: 288
- Total Fat: 22.3g
- Saturated Fat: 8.5g
- Trans Fat: 0g
- Cholesterol: 80mg
- Sodium: 170mg
- Potassium: 62mg
- Total Carb: 2g
- Dietary Fiber: 1.3g
- Sugars: 0.2g
- Protein: 20.6g

Beef Casserole with Asparagus

Serving: 4

Ingredients:

- 1 – pound beef
- 1/4 – Cup chopped onion
- One-teaspoon pepper
- One-teaspoon nutmeg
- 5 – organic eggs
- Two-tablespoons chopped leek
- One-teaspoon paprika
- Half-handful roasted asparagus

Instructions:

- Pour water into the Instant Pot then place a trivet in it.
- Prepare an oven-safe dish then coat with cooking spray.
- Cut the beef into thin slices then place in the prepared dish. Set aside.
- Crack the eggs then chopped onion, pepper, nutmeg, leek, and paprika into the eggs. Whisk until incorporated.
- Pour the egg mixture over the beef then place the dish on the trivet.
- Cover the Instant Pot and seal it properly.
- Select the *Manual* setting then cooks for 30 minutes.
- When the Instant Pot beeps, naturally release it and open the lid.
- Take the dish out from the Instant pot then transfers the casserole to a serving dish.

* Enjoy with roasted asparagus.

Nutrition Info Per Serving:

* Calories: 307
* Total Fat: 13.5g
* Saturated Fat: 4.5g
* Trans Fat: 0g
* Cholesterol: 306mg
* Sodium: 172mg
* Potassium: 567mg
* Total Carb: 2.8g
* Dietary Fiber: 0.9g
* Sugars: 1g
* Protein: 41.9g

Instant Beef Curry

Serving: 4

Ingredients:

* 1 – pound chopped beef chunks
* Two-cloves garlic
* Two-shallots
* Two-tablespoons cayenne pepper
* One-teaspoon turmeric
* One-teaspoon curry powder
* One-teaspoon avocado oil
* One-Cup water
* Half-Cup coconut milk

Instructions:

* Place garlic, shallots, cayenne pepper, turmeric, and curry powder in a food processor. Process until smooth.
* Select the *sauté* setting in an Instant Pot then pours avocado oil into it.
* Stir in spices mixture into the pot then sauté until aromatic. Press the cancel button.
* Add the beef into the Instant Pot then pour water and coconut milk over the beef.
* Cover the Instant Pot with the lid and seal it properly.
* Select the *manual* menu then cook on high for 20 minutes.
* Once it is done, quick release the Instant pot then open the lid.

- Transfer to a serving dish then sprinkles fried shallots on top, if you desired.

Nutrition Info Per Serving:

- Calories: 299
- Total Fat: 15g
- Saturated Fat: 9.2g
- Trans Fat: 0g
- Cholesterol: 101mg
- Sodium: 83mg
- Potassium: 638mg
- Total Carb: 5.2g
- Dietary Fiber: 1.8g
- Sugars: 1.3g
- Protein: 35.8g

Keto Beef Tomato Steak

Serving: 4

Ingredients:

- Two-pounds beef tenderloin
- One-tablespoon chopped onion
- Half-teaspoon nutmeg
- Half-teaspoon pepper
- Two-tablespoons avocado oil
- Half-Cup low sodium beef broth
- One-teaspoon avocado oil
- Two-tablespoons tomato puree
- One-teaspoon paprika

Instructions:

- Cut the beef tenderloin into thick slices
- Combine nutmeg and pepper in a bowl then mixes well.
- Rub the sliced beef with the spices mixture then marinates for at least an hour.
- After an hour, place the seasoned beef into the Instant Pot then pours beef broth into the pot.
- Cover the Instant Pot with the lid and seals it properly.
- Select the *manual* menu then cooks on high for 30 minutes.
- Once it is done, quick release the Instant pot then opens the lid.

- Transfer the cooked beef to a plate then sets aside.

- Select the *Sauté* setting again then pours avocado oil into it.

- Once it is hot, stir the tomato puree and paprika into the pot then mixes until incorporated.

- Return the cooked beef back to the Instant Pot then mixes until combined.

Nutrition Info Per Serving:

- Calories: 499
- Total Fat: 23.1g
- Saturated Fat: 8.3g
- Trans Fat: 0g
- Cholesterol: 209mg
- Sodium: 232mg

- Potassium: 912mg
- Total Carb: 2g
- Dietary Fiber: 0.8g
- Sugars: 0.7g
- Protein: 66.7g

Yummy Mushroom with Beef

Serving: 4

Ingredients:

- 1 – pound beef chunks
- Half-Cup chopped mushroom
- Two-teaspoons sliced shallots
- Half-teaspoon nutmeg
- One-teaspoon pepper
- Half-teaspoon ginger

- One-teaspoon avocado oil
- Two-tablespoons low sodium soy sauce
- One-tablespoon tomato sauce
- Half-Cup low sodium beef broth
- Two-tablespoons chopped carrots

Instructions:

- Place all of the ingredients in an Instant Pot then covers the Instant Pot with the lid and seals it properly.

- Select the *manual* menu then cook on high for 20 minutes.

- When the Instant Pot beeps, quick release the Instant pot then opens the lid.
- Transfer to a serving dish together with the gravy.

Nutrition Info Per Serving:

- Calories: 219
- Total Fat: 7.4g
- Saturated Fat: 2.2g
- Trans Fat: 0g
- Cholesterol: 89mg
- Sodium: 777mg
- Potassium: 114mg
- Total Carb: 2.7g
- Dietary Fiber: 0.6g
- Sugars: 0.8g
- Protein: 35.4g

Beef Roulade in Curry Gravy

Serving: 4

Ingredients:

- Two-pounds beef tenderloin
- Half-teaspoon nutmeg
- Half-teaspoon pepper
- Two-teaspoons minced garlic
- Two-teaspoons sliced shallots
- One-teaspoon turmeric
- Half-teaspoon coriander
- Half-teaspoon black pepper
- One-teaspoon avocado oil
- One-Cup water
- Half-Cup coconut milk

Instructions:

- Cut the beef tenderloin into thin slices
- Combine nutmeg and pepper in a bowl then mixes well.
- Rub the sliced beef with the spices mixture then marinates for at least an hour.
- After an hour, roll the sliced beef then prick each roll using a wooden skewer.
- Pour water into the Instant Pot then place a trivet in it.

- Place the rolled beef on the trivet then covers the Instant Pot with the lid and seals it properly.
- Select the *manual* menu then cooks on high for 30 minutes.
- Once it is done, quick release the Instant pot then opens the lid.
- Take the rolled beef out from the Instant Pot then place on a plate.
- Remove the trivet and discard water from the Instant Pot.
- Select the *sauté* setting in an Instant Pot then pours avocado oil into it.
- Stir in the minced garlic and sliced shallots into the pot then sauté until aromatic. Press the cancel button.
- Add the rolled beef into the Instant Pot then season with turmeric, coriander, and black pepper.
- Pour water and coconut milk over the beef then covers the Instant Pot with the lid and seal it properly.
- Select the *manual* menu then cook on high for 10 minutes.
- Once it is done, quick release the Instant pot then open the lid.
- Transfer to a serving dish.

Nutrition Info Per Serving:

- Calories: 297
- Total Fat: 16.4g
- Saturated Fat: 9.9g
- Trans Fat: 0g
- Cholesterol: 90mg
- Sodium: 74mg
- Potassium: 523mg
- Total Carb: 3.1g
- Dietary Fiber: 1g
- Sugars: 1.1g
- Protein: 33.3g

Serving: 6

Ingredients:

- 1 – pound grass-fed beef
- Two-teaspoons minced garlic
- Two-teaspoons sliced shallot
- Three-teaspoons garam masala
- 1/4 – teaspoon paprika
- 1/4 – teaspoon turmeric
- One-teaspoon cayenne
- Two-tablespoons red chili flakes
- Two-kaffir lime leaves
- Two-lemon grasses
- One-inch galangal
- One-Cup low sodium beef broth

Instructions:

- Place garlic, shallots, garam masala, paprika, turmeric, cayenne, and red chili flakes in a food processor. Process until smooth.
- Transfer the spices to an Instant Pot then add the beef in it.
- Add kaffir lime leaves, lemon grasses, and galangal into the Instant Pot then pour beef broth over the beef.
- Cover the Instant Pot with the lid and seal it properly.
- Select the *manual* menu then cook on high for 30 minutes.
- Once it is done, quick release the Instant pot then open the lid.
- Using two forks chop the beef then transfers to a serving dish together with the gravy.
- Serve warm.

Nutrition Info Per Serving:

- Calories: 190
- Total Fat: 13.7g
- Saturated Fat: 5.4g
- Trans Fat: 0g
- Cholesterol: 54mg
- Sodium: 189mg
- Potassium: 75mg
- Total Carb: 2.7g
- Dietary Fiber: 0.2g
- Sugars: 0.4g
- Protein: 14.5g

Serving: 4

Ingredients:

- Two-pounds beef ribs
- Half-Cup tomato paste
- Half-tablespoon Worcestershire sauce
- One-teaspoon smoked paprika
- One-teaspoon minced garlic
- One-tablespoon chopped onion
- 1/4 – teaspoon chili powder
- 1/4 – teaspoon cayenne pepper
- Two-tablespoons avocado oil

Instructions:

- Combine all ingredients except beef in a bowl. Mix until incorporated.
- Rub the beef ribs with the mixture then wraps with aluminum foil.
- Pour water in the Instant Pot then place a trivet in it.
- Place the wrapped beef on the trivet then covers and seals it properly.
- Select the *Manual* setting then cooks for 30 minutes.
- When the Instant Pot beeps, quick release it and open the lid.
- Take the wrapped beef from the Instant pot then unwraps it.
- Transfer to a serving dish.

Nutrition Info Per Serving:

- Calories: 394
- Total Fat: 27.6g
- Saturated Fat: 10.6g
- Trans Fat: 0g
- Cholesterol: 91mg
- Sodium: 117mg
- Potassium: 620mg
- Total Carb: 4.1g
- Dietary Fiber: 0.9g
- Sugars: 2.1g
- Protein: 31g

Serving: 4

Ingredients:

- 3/4 pound 'chuck steak
- One-lemon grass
- Three-shallots
- Four-cloves garlic
- Half-Cup cayenne pepper
- One-teaspoon ginger
- One-inch galangal
- Half-tablespoon avocado oil
- Half-teaspoon cumin
- One-teaspoon coriander
- Half-teaspoon turmeric
- Half-Cup coconut milk
- One-kaffir lime leaf
- One-cinnamon stick
- One-teaspoon tamarind
- One-tablespoon low sodium soy sauce
- Half-teaspoon pepper

Instructions:

- Place shallots, garlic, cayenne pepper, ginger, and galangal in a food processor. Process until smooth.
- Select the *Sauté* setting of an Instant Pot then pours avocado oil into it.
- Once it is hot, stir in the spices mixture then sautés until aromatic.
- Add the beef together with cumin, coriander, turmeric, cinnamon stick, tamarind, pepper, soy sauce, and kaffir lime leaves then stirs until the beef is completely coated.
- Pour coconut milk over the beef then covers the Instant Pot with the lid and seals it properly.
- Select the *manual* menu then cook on high for 30 minutes.
- When the Instant Pot beeps, naturally release the Instant pot then opens the lid.
- Transfer to a serving dish together with the gravy then serves immediately.
- If you want the gravy to be thickened, transfer the beef and gravy to a pan then bring to a simmer until the liquid reduces.

!

Nutrition Info Per Serving:

- Calories: 253
- Total Fat: 19.6g
- Saturated Fat: 11.2g
- Trans Fat: 0g
- Cholesterol: 48mg
- Sodium: 190mg
- Potassium: 274mg
- Total Carb: 6.6g
- Dietary Fiber: 1.6g
- Sugars: 1.6g
- Protein: 13.8g

Awesome Keto Ribs Soup

Serving: 4

Ingredients:

- Two-pounds beef ribs
- Two-teaspoons minced garlic
- One-teaspoon pepper
- One-teaspoon avocado oil
- Three-cups water
- Two-cups chopped collard green

Instructions:

- Select the *Sauté* setting of an Instant Pot then pours avocado oil into it.
- Once it is hot, stir in minced garlic then sautés until brown and aromatic. Press the *Cancel* button.
- Add beef ribs into the pot then pours water into it.
- Season with pepper then covers the Instant pot properly.
- Select the *Manual* setting then cooks on high for 30 minutes.
- When the Instant Pot beeps, quick release the Instant Pot then opens the lid.
- Quickly stir in the chopped collard green then mixes until the vegetable is wilted.
- Transfer to a soup bowl.

Nutrition Info Per Serving:

- Calories: 304
- Total Fat: 13.2g
- Saturated Fat: 4.9g
- Trans Fat: 0g

- Cholesterol: 130mg
- Sodium: 95mg
- Potassium: 537mg
- Total Carb: 2.1g
- Dietary Fiber: 1g
- Sugars: 0g
- Protein: 42g

Keto Brown Beef Tender

Serving: 4

Ingredients:

- 1 – pound beef chunks
- One-teaspoon nutmeg
- Two-teaspoons black pepper
- Two-tablespoons chopped onion
- Two-tablespoons low sodium soy sauce
- Half-cup water

Instructions:

- Place nutmeg, black pepper, chopped onion, and soy sauce in a bowl then mixes until incorporated.
- Rub the beef with the spices mixture then let it sit for at least an hour. If you want to rub it longer, place in a container with a lid then chills in the refrigerator.
- Place the seasoned beef in the Instant Pot then pours water over the beef.
- Cover the Instant Pot with the lid and seals it properly.
- Select the *manual* menu then cook on high for 25 minutes.
- Once the beef is done, naturally release the Instant pot then opens the lid.
- Transfer to a serving dish.

Nutrition Info Per Serving:

- Calories: 223
- Total Fat: 7.3g
- Saturated Fat: 2.8g
- Trans Fat: 0g
- Cholesterol: 101mg
- Sodium: 376mg
- Potassium: 496mg
- Total Carb: 2.2g

- Dietary Fiber: 0.6g
- Sugars: 0.5g
- Protein: 35.1g

Serving: 4

Ingredients:

- 1 – pound ground beef
- 1/4 – Cup almond flour
- One-organic egg
- One-tablespoon minced garlic
- One-teaspoon pepper
- One-Cup low sodium beef broth

Instructions:

- Place the ground beef in a food processor together with almond flour, egg, and minced garlic. Process until smooth.
- Shape the beef mixture into logs then wrap each log with aluminum foil.
- Pour beef broth into the Instant Pot then place a trivet in it.
- Place the wrapped logs on the trivet then covers and seals it properly.
- Select the *Manual* setting then cooks for 20 minutes.
- When the Instant Pot beeps, naturally release it and open the lid.
- Take the logs out from the Instant pot then unwraps them.
- Arrange on a serving dish and serve with fresh green and lemon.

!

Nutrition Info Per Serving:

- Calories: 281
- Total Fat: 12g
- Saturated Fat: 3.4g
- Trans Fat: 0g
- Cholesterol: 142mg
- Sodium: 281mg
- Potassium: 538mg
- Total Carb: 2.8g
- Dietary Fiber: 0.9g
- Sugars: 0.5g
- Protein: 38.7g

Serving: 4

Ingredients:

- Two-pounds beef chuck roast
- 3/4 – teaspoon black pepper
- Two-teaspoons minced garlic
- 1 and ½ – tablespoons coconut oil
- 1/4 – Cup chopped onion
- 1 and ½ – cups low sodium beef broth

Instructions:

- Cut the beef into thick slices then rub with black pepper and minced garlic.
- Select the *Sauté* setting of an Instant Pot then pours coconut oil into it.
- Once it is hot, stir in chopped onion into the Instant Pot then sautés until wilted and aromatic.
- Add the beef into the pot then pours beef broth over the beef.
- Cover the Instant Pot with the lid and seal it properly.
- Select the *manual* menu then cooks on high for 40 minutes.
- Once it is done, quick release the Instant pot then opens the lid.
- Transfer the cooked beef to a plate.

!

Nutrition Info Per Serving:

- Calories: 282
- Total Fat: 15.4g
- Saturated Fat: 8.3g
- Trans Fat: 0g
- Cholesterol: 83mg
- Sodium: 273mg
- Potassium: 494mg
- Total Carb: 1.6g
- Dietary Fiber: 0.3g
- Sugars: 0.5g
- Protein: 32.4g

Serving: 4

Ingredients:

- 1 – pound beef tenderloin
- One-teaspoon avocado oil
- One-onion, cut into quarters
- One-teaspoon minced garlic
- Two-tablespoons red chili flakes
- One-teaspoon pepper
- Two-tablespoons low sodium soy sauce
- 1/4 – Cup water
- One-teaspoon chopped celery

Instructions:

- Select the *Sauté* setting in an Instant Pot then pours avocado oil into it.
- Add the quartered onion, minced garlic, and red chili flakes into the pot then sautés until aromatic and brown. Press the *Cancel* button.
- Cut the beef tenderloin into thin slices then add them into the pot.
- Season with pepper then drizzle the low sodium soy sauce over the beef.
- Pour water into the pot then covers the Instant Pot with the lid and seals it properly.
- Select the *manual* menu then cook on high for 30 minutes.
- Once it is done, quick release the Instant pot then open the lid.
- Transfer to a serving dish together with the liquid then sprinkles chopped celeries on top.

Nutrition Info Per Serving:

- Calories: 255
- Total Fat: 10.6g
- Saturated Fat: 4g
- Trans Fat: 0g
- Cholesterol: 104mg
- Sodium: 370mg
- Potassium: 491mg
- Total Carb: 4.4g
- Dietary Fiber: 0.9g
- Sugars: 1.6g
- Protein: 33.8g

Serving: 4

Ingredients:

- 1 – pound beef
- One-tablespoon minced garlic
- One-teaspoon pepper
- 1/4 – Cup tomato puree
- Two-tablespoons tomato sauce
- Two-teaspoons avocado oil

Instructions:

- Combine minced garlic with pepper, tomato puree, tomato sauce, and avocado oil in a bowl. Mix until incorporated.
- Dip the beef in the spices mixture and make sure that the beef is completely coated with the spices.
- Wrap the beef with aluminum foil then sets aside.
- Pour water in the Instant Pot then place a trivet in it.
- Place the wrapped beef on the trivet then covers and seals it properly.
- Select the *Manual* setting then cooks for 30 minutes.
- When the Instant Pot beeps, naturally release it and open the lid.
- Take the wrapped beef from the Instant pot then unwraps it.
- Transfer to a serving dish and garnish with any kinds of green, as you desired.

Nutrition Info Per Serving:

- Calories: 226
- Total Fat: 7.4g
- Saturated Fat: 2.7g
- Trans Fat: 0g
- Cholesterol: 101mg
- Sodium: 120mg
- Potassium: 573mg
- Total Carb: 3g
- Dietary Fiber: 0.7g
- Sugars: 1.1g
- Protein: 35g

Serving: 4

Ingredients:

- 1 – pound beef chunks
- 1/4 – Cup chopped onion
- One-teaspoon pepper
- One-teaspoon avocado oil
- Two-tablespoons low sodium soy sauce
- One-tablespoon tomato sauce
- One-Cup low sodium beef broth
- 1/4 – Cup broccoli florets
- 1/4 – Cup cauliflower florets
- Two-tablespoons chopped carrots

Instructions:

- Select the *sauté* setting in an Instant Pot then pours avocado oil into it.
- Stir in the chopped onion into the pot then sauté until aromatic. Press the cancel button.
- Add the beef chunks into the Instant Pot then season pepper.
- Drizzle tomato sauce and soy sauce over the beef then add carrots into the pot.
- Pour beef broth over the beef then covers the Instant Pot with the lid and seal it properly.
- Select the *manual* menu then cook on high for 20 minutes.
- Once it is done, quick release the Instant pot then opens the lid.
- Add broccoli and cauliflower into the pot then stirs until the vegetable is wilted.
- Transfer to a serving dish then serves immediately.

Nutrition Info Per Serving:

- Calories: 64
- Total Fat: 3.3g
- Saturated Fat: 1.3g
- Trans Fat: 0g
- Cholesterol: 9mg
- Sodium: 262mg
- Potassium: 157mg
- Total Carb: 5.7g
- Dietary Fiber: 1.5g
- Sugars: 1.3g
- Protein: 3.2g

Serving: 4

Ingredients:

- 1 – pound grass-fed beef
- 1/4 – Cup chopped onion
- Half-teaspoon nutmeg
- Half-teaspoon black pepper
- One-teaspoon avocado oil
- 1/4 – Cup low sodium beef broth
- 1/4 – Cup chopped red tomatoes
- 1/4 – Cup chopped cucumber

Instructions:

- Cut the beef into thin slices then sets aside.
- Select the *Sauté* setting in an Instant Pot then pours avocado oil into it.
- Once it is hot, stir in chopped onion then sautés until aromatic. Press the cancel button.
- Add the sliced beef into the Instant Pot then seasons with nutmeg and black pepper.
- Pour water over the beef then covers the Instant Pot with the lid and seal it properly.
- Select the *manual* menu then cook on high for 30 minutes.
- Once it is done, quick release the Instant pot then open the lid.
- Arrange chopped tomatoes and cucumber on a serving platter then add the cooked beef on top.

Nutrition Info Per Serving:

- Calories: 273
- Total Fat: 20.5g
- Saturated Fat: 8.2g
- Trans Fat: 0g
- Cholesterol: 80mg
- Sodium: 129mg
- Potassium: 68mg
- Total Carb: 1.8g
- Dietary Fiber: 0.5g
- Sugars: 0.8g
- Protein: 20.7g

Serving: 4

Ingredients:

- 1 – pound grass-fed beef
- Two-tablespoons chopped onion
- One-teaspoon avocado oil
- Three-tablespoons low sodium soy sauce
- One-teaspoon pepper
- One-teaspoon nutmeg
- Three-cups water

Instructions:

- Select the *sauté* setting in an Instant Pot then pours avocado oil into it.
- Stir in the chopped onion into the pot then sauté until aromatic. Press the cancel button.
- Cut the beef into slices then add them into the Instant Pot.
- Sprinkle pepper and nutmeg then drizzle soy sauce over the beef.
- Pour water into the Instant Pot then covers the Instant Pot with the lid and seal it properly.
- Select the *manual* menu then cook on high for 30 minutes.
- Once it is done, quick release the Instant pot then open the lid.
- Transfer to a serving dish.

Nutrition Info Per Serving:

- Calories: 177
- Total Fat: 6.5g
- Saturated Fat: 2.2g
- Trans Fat: 0g
- Cholesterol: 41mg
- Sodium: 517mg
- Potassium: 441mg
- Total Carb: 2.3g
- Dietary Fiber: 0.5g
- Sugars: 0.6g
- Protein: 26.2g

Serving: 6

Ingredients:

- 1 – pound grass-fed beef
- One-teaspoon nutmeg
- Half-teaspoon pepper
- 1/4 – Cup chopped onion
- One-Cup tomato puree
- Two-tablespoons tomato paste
- One-medium tomato
- One-Cup low sodium beef broth

Instructions:

- Cut the beef into thick slices then place in an Instant Pot.
- Season with nutmeg, pepper, and onion.
- Cut the tomato
- Place garlic, shallots, garam masala, paprika, turmeric, cayenne, and red chili flakes in a food processor. Process until smooth.
- Transfer the spices to an Instant Pot then add the beef in it.
- Add kaffir lime leaves, lemon grasses, and galangal into the Instant Pot then pour beef broth over the beef.
- Cover the Instant Pot with the lid and seal it properly.
- Select the *manual* menu then cook on high for 30 minutes.
- Once it is done, quick release the Instant pot then open the lid.
- Using two forks chop the beef then transfers to a serving dish together with the gravy.
- Serve warm.

Nutrition Info Per Serving:

- Calories: 209
- Total Fat: 13.9g
- Saturated Fat: 5.5g
- Trans Fat: 0g
- Cholesterol: 54mg
- Sodium: 199mg
- Potassium: 331mg
- Total Carb: 6.5g
- Dietary Fiber: 1.5g
- Sugars: 3.6g
- Protein: 15.4g

Keto Chicken Balls

Serving: 4

Ingredients:

- 1 – pound ground chicken
- Half-Cup almond flour
- Two-organic eggs
- 1/4 – teaspoon pepper
- One-teaspoon minced garlic
- Two-tablespoons diced onion
- 1/4 – teaspoon oregano
- Half-Cup low sodium chicken broth
- Half-Cup tomato puree

Instructions:

- Place the ground chicken in a bowl then add almond flour into the bowl.
- Season with pepper, minced garlic, diced onion, and oregano then adds the eggs over the chicken.
- Using your hand, mix the ingredients then shape into medium ball forms. Set aside.
- Pour water and tomato puree into an Instant pot then stir well.
- Add the balls into the Instant Pot then cover and seal it properly.
- Select the *Manual* setting then cooks for 10 minutes.
- When the Instant Pot beeps, naturally release it and open the lid.
- Transfer the chicken balls to a serving dish together with the gravy.

Nutrition Info Per Serving:

- Calories: 284
- Total Fat: 18.4g
- Saturated Fat: 3.8g
- Trans Fat: 0.1g
- Cholesterol: 179mg
- Sodium: 108mg
- Potassium: 635mg
- Total Carb: 5.2g
- Dietary Fiber: 1.8g
- Sugars: 0.9g
- Protein: 26.2g

Serving: 6

Ingredients:

- 1 – pound chopped organic chicken

For The Marinate:

- Half-Cup plain yogurt
- Three-teaspoons garam masala
- Three-teaspoons lemon juice
- One-teaspoon pepper
- 1/4 – teaspoon ginger

For The Sauce:

- 3/4 – cup tomato puree
- Two-teaspoons minced garlic
- Three-teaspoons garam masala
- 1/4 – teaspoon paprika
- 1/4 – teaspoon turmeric
- 1/4 – teaspoon cayenne
- One-Cup heavy cream

Instructions:

- Combine plain yogurt, garam masala, lemon juice, pepper, and ginger in a bowl then mix well.
- Rub the chicken with the spices mixture then marinates for about an hour.
- After an hour, choose the *sauté* mode on an Instant Pot then stir in the chicken. Sauté until the chicken is no longer pink.
- Add the remaining spices mixture into the Instant Pot together with tomato puree, minced garlic, garam masala, paprika, turmeric, and cayenne.
- Cover the Instant Pot with the lid and seal it properly.
- Select the *manual* menu then cook on high for 10 minutes.

- Once it is done, quick release the Instant pot then open the lid.
- Select the *sauté* menu again then pours heavy cream over the chicken. Stir until the gravy is thickened then transfers to a serving dish.
- Serve warm.

Nutrition Info Per Serving:

- Calories: 214
- Total Fat: 10.1g
- Saturated Fat: 5.5g
- Trans Fat: 0g
- Cholesterol: 87mg
- Sodium: 81mg
- Potassium: 360mg
- Total Carb: 5.6g
- Dietary Fiber: 0.8g
- Sugars: 3.1g
- Protein: 24.2g

Special Keto Chicken Soup

Serving: 4

Ingredients:

- 1 – pound organic chicken breast
- Two-cups low sodium vegetable stock
- Two-lemon grasses
- One-inch galangal
- Two-kaffir lime leaves
- Two-teaspoons red chili flakes
- One-teaspoon red chili paste
- 1/4 – Cup chopped red tomatoes
- One-tablespoon sliced shallot
- Two-tablespoons lemon juice
- One-teaspoon cilantro

Instructions:

- Cut the chicken into cubes then place in an Instant Pot.
- Add the remaining ingredients into the pot then covers with the lid.
- Seal the pot properly then selects the *manual* menu and cooks on high for 15 minutes.
- Once it is done, quick release the Instant pot then open the lid.
- Transfer to a serving dish then garnish with fresh celery on top.

Nutrition Info Per Serving:

- Calories: 158
- Total Fat: 3.2g

- Saturated Fat: 0.1g
- Trans Fat: 0g
- Cholesterol: 73mg
- Sodium: 153mg
- Potassium: 555mg
- Total Carb: 6g
- Dietary Fiber: 0.8g
- Sugars: 2.5g
- Protein: 24.9g

Classic Keto Buttery Chicken Wings

Serving: 4

Ingredients:

- 1 – pound organic chicken wings
- One-Cup water
- Two-tablespoons lemon juice
- One-tablespoon butter
- One-tablespoon tomato sauce

Instructions:

- Pour water into an Instant Pot then place a trivet in it.
- Rub the chicken with lemon juice then place the chicken on the prepared trivet.
- Cover the Instant Pot with the lid and seal it properly.
- Select the *manual* menu then cook on high for 10 minutes.
- Meanwhile, place butter and tomato sauce in a microwave–safe bowl then microwave on low until melted.
- Once the chicken is done, quick release the Instant pot then open the lid.
- Transfer the chicken to bowl then drizzle melted butter on it.
- Shake until the chicken is completely coated with butter then serve.

Nutrition Info Per Serving:

- Calories: 244
- Total Fat: 11.4g
- Saturated Fat: 4.2g
- Trans Fat: 0g
- Sodium: 141mg
- Potassium: 299mg
- Total Carb: 0.4g
- Dietary Fiber: 0.1g
- Sugars: 0.3g
- Protein: 33g

Serving: 4

Ingredients:

- 1 – pound organic boneless chicken
- Two-lemon grasses
- Two-teaspoons minced garlic
- One-teaspoon ginger
- 3/4 – cup coconut milk
- Half-teaspoon black pepper
- One-teaspoon avocado oil
- 1/4 – Cup chopped onion
- One-tablespoon lemon juice

Instructions:

- Rub the chicken with lemon juice then sets aside.
- Cut the melon grasses into thin slices then place in a bowl.
- Select the *sauté* setting in an Instant Pot then pours avocado oil into it.
- Once it is hot, stir in sliced lemon grasses, chopped onion, and minced garlic into the pot then sauté until aromatic. Press the cancel button.
- Add the chicken into the Instant Pot then seasons with ginger and black pepper.
- Pour coconut milk over the chicken then covers the Instant Pot with the lid and seal it properly.
- Select the *manual* menu then cook on high for 25 minutes.
- Once it is done, quick release the Instant pot then open the lid.
- Transfer to a serving dish then garnish with any kinds of vegetables, as you desired.

Nutrition Info Per Serving:

- Calories: 331
- Total Fat: 19.4g
- Saturated Fat: 11.9g
- Trans Fat: 0g
- Cholesterol: 101mg
- Sodium: 106mg
- Potassium: 445mg
- Total Carb: 4.9g
- Dietary Fiber: 1.4g
- Sugars: 1.9g
- Protein: 34.2g

Serving: 4

Ingredients:

- 1-organic whole chicken
- One-tablespoon avocado oil
- 1 and ½ – teaspoons paprika
- 1 and ½ – cup low sodium chicken broth
- One-teaspoon thyme
- Half-teaspoon black pepper
- Two-tablespoons lemon juice
- 1/4 – Cup minced garlic

Instructions:

- Choose the medium chicken—about 4 lbs.
- Drizzle lemon juice over the chicken then let it sit for about 5 minutes.
- Meanwhile, place paprika, thyme, black pepper, and garlic in a bowl. Mix until combined.
- Rub the chicken with the spices mixture then squeezes until the chicken is completely seasoned.
- Select *Sauté* setting in an Instant pot then pours avocado oil into it.
- Add the chicken into the pot then sauté for about 5 minutes then flips the chicken.
- Pour chicken broth over the chicken then covers the Instant Pot with the lid and seals it properly.
- Select the *manual* menu then cooks on high for 25 minutes.
- Once it is done, quick release the Instant pot then opens the lid.
- Transfer the chicken to a serving dish.
- Serve warm.

Nutrition Info Per Serving:

- Calories: 448
- Total Fat: 28.7g
- Saturated Fat: 8.2g
- Trans Fat: 0g
- Cholesterol: 190mg
- Sodium: 210mg
- Total Carb: 4.3g
- Dietary Fiber: 0.8g
- Sugars: 0.3g
- Protein: 41.6g

Serving: 4

Ingredients:

- 1 – pound organic chicken fillet
- Half-teaspoon pepper
- 1/4 – teaspoon nutmeg
- Two-tablespoons sesame oil
- Two-tablespoons lemon juice
- One-tablespoon sesame seeds

Instructions:

- Select the *Sauté* setting in an Instant Pot then pour sesame oil into it.
- Add the chicken into the pot then browns each side of the chicken. Press the cancel button.
- Drizzle lemon juice over the chicken then seasons with pepper and nutmeg.
- Cover the Instant Pot then seals it properly.
- Select the *manual* setting then cooks on high for 5 minutes.
- Once it is done, quick release the Instant Pot then opens the lid.
- Transfer to a serving dish then sprinkles sesame seeds on top.
- Serves immediately.

Nutrition Info Per Serving:

- Calories: 292
- Total Fat: 16.4g
- Saturated Fat: 3.5g
- Trans Fat: 0g
- Cholesterol: 101mg
- Sodium: 99mg
- Potassium: 299mg
- Total Carb: 0.9g
- Dietary Fiber: 0.4g
- Sugars: 0.2g
- Protein: 33.3g

Serving: 6

Ingredients:

- 1 – pound chopped organic chicken
- Two-teaspoons minced garlic
- Two-teaspoons sliced shallot
- One-teaspoon paprika
- 1/4 – teaspoon turmeric
- 1/4 – teaspoon cayenne
- 1 and ½ – teaspoons red chili flakes
- Half-Cup water
- One-Cup coconut milk

Instructions:

- Combine garlic, shallot, paprika, turmeric, cayenne, and red chili flakes in a food processor. Process until smooth then set aside.
- Place chopped chicken in an Instant Pot then add the spices mixture over the chicken.
- Pour water over the chicken then covers the Instant Pot with the lid and seal it properly.
- Select the *manual* menu then cook on high for 10 minutes.
- Once it is done, quick release the Instant pot then open the lid.
- Select the *sauté* menu again then pour coconut milk over the chicken. Stir until the gravy is thickened then transfers to a serving dish.
- Serve warm.

Nutrition Info Per Serving:

- Calories: 277
- Total Fat: 23.2g
- Saturated Fat: 13.9g
- Trans Fat: 0g
- Cholesterol: 54mg
- Sodium: 190mg
- Potassium: 162mg
- Total Carb: 3.4g
- Dietary Fiber: 1.1g
- Sugars: 1.5g
- Protein: 15.3g

Serving: 4

Ingredients:

- 1 – pound organic chicken thighs
- Two-tablespoons sliced shallots
- One-teaspoon ginger
- One-teaspoon pepper
- One-teaspoon nutmeg
- Four-Cups water
- One-tablespoon leek

Instructions:

- Place chicken and all of the ingredients except chopped leek in an Instant Pot.
- Pour water over the chicken then covers the Instant Pot with the lid and seal it properly.
- Select the *manual* menu then cook on high for 25 minutes.
- Once it is done, quick release the Instant pot then open the lid.
- Transfer to a serving dish then garnish with chopped leek on top.
- Serve Warm!

!

Nutrition Info Per Serving:

- Calories: 226
- Total Fat: 8.7g
- Saturated Fat: 2.5g
- Trans Fat: 0g
- Cholesterol: 101mg
- Sodium: 106mg
- Potassium: 312mg
- Total Carb: 2g
- Dietary Fiber: 0.3g
- Sugars: 0.2g
- Protein: 33.1g

Serving: 4

Ingredients:

- 1 – pound organic chopped chicken
- Two-tablespoons lemon juice
- 1/4 – Cup diced red tomato
- Two-cups fresh basil
- 1/4 – Cup chopped leek
- One-teaspoon avocado oil
- Four-shallots
- 5 – cloves garlic
- One-teaspoon turmeric
- One-teaspoon ginger
- Two-candlenuts
- 1/4 – Cup cayenne pepper
- Three-lemon grasses
- Two-kaffir lime leaves
- One-Cup hot water

Instructions:

- Rub the chicken with lemon juice then let it sit for about 20 minutes.
- Meanwhile, place shallots, garlic, turmeric, ginger, candlenuts, and chili in a food processor. Process until smooth then sets aside.
- After 20 minutes, select the *sauté* setting in an Instant Pot then pours avocado oil into it.
- Stir in the spices mixture then sautés until aromatic.
- Add lemon grasses and kaffir lime leaves into the pot then sautés until wilted.
- Place the chicken in the Instant Pot then mixes with the spices until the chicken is completely seasoned. Press the *Cancel* button.
- Pour water over the chicken then covers the Instant Pot with the lid and seal it properly.
- Select the *manual* menu then cook on high for 15 minutes.
- Once it is done, quick release the Instant pot then open the lid.
- Quickly add diced tomato, fresh basils, and chopped leeks into the pot then stir until the vegetables are wilted.
- Transfer to a serving dish.

Nutrition Info Per Serving:

- Calories: 86
- Total Fat: 3.3g
- Saturated Fat: 0.3g
- Trans Fat: 0g
- Cholesterol: 18mg
- Sodium: 26mg
- Potassium: 291mg
- Total Carb: 6.9g
- Dietary Fiber: 1.2g
- Sugars: 0.9g
- Protein: 7.7g

Healthy Chicken Curry Soup

Serving: 4

Ingredients:

- 1 – pound chopped organic chicken
- Two-teaspoons minced garlic
- Two-teaspoons sliced shallots
- One-teaspoon turmeric
- Half-teaspoon coriander
- Half-teaspoon pepper
- One-teaspoon avocado oil
- One-Cup water
- Half-Cup coconut milk
- One-green tomato

Instructions:

- Select the *sauté* setting in an Instant Pot then pours avocado oil into it.
- Stir in the minced garlic and sliced shallots into the pot then sauté until aromatic. Press the cancel button.
- Add the chicken into the Instant Pot then season with turmeric, coriander, and pepper.
- Pour water and coconut milk over the chicken then covers the Instant Pot with the lid and seal it properly.
- Select the *manual* menu then cook on high for 20 minutes.
- Once it is done, quick release the Instant pot then open the lid.
- Cut the green tomatoes into quarters then add into the pot. Stir until the tomatoes are wilted.
- Transfer to a serving.

Nutrition Info Per Serving:

- Calories: 214
- Total Fat: 10.1g

- Saturated Fat: 5.5g
- Trans Fat: 0g
- Cholesterol: 87mg
- Sodium: 81mg
- Potassium: 360mg
- Total Carb: 5.6g
- Dietary Fiber: 0.8g
- Sugars: 3.1g
- Protein: 24.2g

Awesome Keto Shredded Chicken

Serving: 4

Ingredients:

- 1 – pound organic boneless chicken
- One-teaspoon minced garlic
- 1/4 – teaspoon pepper
- 1/4 – teaspoon cumin
- 1/4 – teaspoon smoked paprika
- One-Cup low sodium chicken broth

Instructions:

- Place all ingredients in an Instant Pot.
- Cover the pot with its lid then seals it properly.
- Select the *manual* setting then cooks on high for 20 minutes.
- Once the Instant Pot beeps, quick release the Instant Pot then opens the lid.
- Using two forks, shred the cooked chicken into pieces then transfers to a serving dish.

Nutrition Info Per Serving:

- Calories: 221
- Total Fat: 8.5g
- Saturated Fat: 2.3g
- Trans Fat: 0g
- Cholesterol: 101mg
- Sodium: 115mg
- Potassium: 285mg
- Total Carb: 0.7g
- Dietary Fiber: 0.1g
- Sugars: 0g
- Protein: 33.4g

Serving: 4

Ingredients:

- 1 – pound organic chicken fillet
- Half-Cup chopped mushroom
- One-teaspoon avocado oil
- Two-tablespoons chopped onion
- 4 – whole shallots
- One-teaspoon pepper
- Half-teaspoon nutmeg
- Two-tablespoons low sodium soy sauce
- Half-Cup low sodium chicken broth

Instructions:

- Select the *Sauté* setting in an Instant Pot then pours avocado oil into it.
- Add the chopped onion then sautés until aromatic and brown. Press the *Cancel* button.
- Stir in the chicken fillet together with the remaining ingredients.
- After that, cover the Instant Pot with the lid and seal it properly.
- Select the *manual* menu then cook on high for 10 minutes.
- Once it is done, quick release the Instant pot then open the lid.
- Transfer to a serving dish.

Nutrition Info Per Serving:

- Calories: 238
- Total Fat: 8.7g
- Saturated Fat: 2.4g
- Trans Fat: 0g
- Cholesterol: 101mg
- Sodium: 408mg
- Potassium: 372mg
- Total Carb: 3.9g
- Dietary Fiber: 0.5g
- Sugars: 0.6g
- Protein: 34.2g

Serving: 4

Ingredients:

- 1 – pound organic chicken wings
- Two-teaspoons minced garlic
- One-teaspoon pepper
- One-teaspoon nutmeg
- Two-tablespoons avocado oil
- One-Cup water
- 1/4 – Cup tomato sauce
- One-teaspoon paprika

Instructions:

- Pour water into an Instant Pot then place a trivet in it.
- Combine minced garlic, pepper, nutmeg, and avocado oil in a bowl then mixes until incorporated.
- Rub the chicken with the spices mixture then place the chicken on the prepared trivet.
- Cover the Instant Pot with the lid and seal it properly.
- Select the *manual* menu then cook on high for 10 minutes.
- Meanwhile, place tomato sauce in a microwave–safe bowl then microwave on low until warm.
- Add paprika into the warmed tomato sauce then mix until incorporated.
- Once the chicken is done, quick release the Instant pot then open the lid.
- Transfer the chicken to bowl with tomato sauce then stirs until the chicken is completely coated with tomato sauce.
- Arrange the chicken on a serving dish.

Nutrition Info Per Serving:

- Calories: 236
- Total Fat: 9.6g
- Saturated Fat: 2.7g
- Trans Fat: 0g
- Cholesterol: 101mg
- Sodium: 181mg
- Potassium: 376mg
- Total Carb: 2.6g
- Dietary Fiber: 1g
- Sugars: 0.9g
- Protein: 33.4g

Serving: 4

Ingredients:

- 1 – pound organic chicken fillet
- Two-teaspoons minced garlic
- Two-teaspoons sliced shallots
- One-tablespoons red chili flakes
- One-teaspoon paprika
- Two-teaspoons cayenne
- 5 – kaffir lime leaves
- Two-tablespoons tomato puree
- One-Cup water
- One-Cup broccoli florets

Instructions:

- Cut the chicken fillet into cubes then place in an Instant Pot.
- Add the remaining ingredients except for broccoli florets into the pot then cover the Instant Pot with the lid and seal it properly.
- Select the *manual* menu then cook on high for 10 minutes.
- Once it is done, quick release the Instant pot then open the lid.
- Stir in the broccoli florets then stirs until wilted.
- Transfer to a serving dish.

Nutrition Info Per Serving:

- Calories: 247
- Total Fat: 8.8g
- Saturated Fat: 2.4g
- Trans Fat: 0g
- Cholesterol: 101mg
- Sodium: 129mg
- Potassium: 432mg
- Total Carb: 7.7g
- Dietary Fiber: 1.3g
- Sugars: 1g
- Protein: 33.9g

Serving: 4

Ingredients:

- 4 – pounds organic bone in chicken
- 1 and ½ – tablespoons sliced garlic
- One-tablespoon ginger
- Four-Cups low sodium chicken broth
- One-tablespoon avocado oil

Instructions:

- Place the chicken in an Instant Pot then sprinkles sliced garlic and ginger over the chicken.
- Pour chicken broth into the Instant Pot then covers the Instant Pot properly.
- Select the *manual* setting and cook for 15 minutes.
- Once the chicken is done, quick release the Instant Pot then opens the lid.
- Quickly drizzle avocado oil over the chicken then mixes well.
- Transfer to a serving dish then serves.

!

Nutrition Info Per Serving:

- Calories: 105
- Total Fat: 0.5g
- Saturated Fat: 0.1g
- Trans Fat: 0g
- Cholesterol: 0mg
- Sodium: 865mg
- Potassium: 42mg
- Total Carb: 3.2g
- Dietary Fiber: 0.4g
- Sugars: 0.1g
- Protein: 19.4g

Serving: 4

Ingredients:

- 1 – pound organic chicken breast
- One-teaspoon minced garlic
- One-teaspoon black pepper
- One-teaspoon paprika
- Two-tablespoons avocado oil
- Two-tablespoons lemon juice
- One-Cup low sodium chicken broth

Instructions:

- Combine minced garlic, paprika, black pepper, lemon juice, and avocado oil in a bowl. Mix well.
- Rub the chicken with the spices mixture then marinates for about an hour.
- After an hour, choose the *sauté* mode on an Instant Pot then stir in the chicken. Sauté until the chicken is crisp and no longer pink.
- Take the chicken out from the Instant Pot then place in a plate.
- Place a trivet in the Instant Pot then pours chicken broth into the pot.
- Return the chicken back into the Instant Pot then place on the trivet.
- Cover the Instant Pot with the lid and seals it properly.
- Select the *manual* menu then cooks on high for 20 minutes.
- Once it is done, quick release the Instant pot then opens the lid.
- Transfer the chicken to a serving dish.
- Serve warm.

Nutrition Info Per Serving:

- Calories: 148
- Total Fat: 3.9g
- Saturated Fat: 0.3g
- Trans Fat: 0g
- Cholesterol: 73mg
- Sodium: 78mg
- Potassium: 473mg
- Total Carb: 1.7g
- Dietary Fiber: 0.7g
- Sugars: 0.2g
- Protein: 24.9g

Serving: 4

Ingredients:

- 1 – pound chopped organic chicken breast
- Two-teaspoons minced garlic
- Two-tablespoons sliced shallots
- One-tablespoon green chili flakes
- One-tablespoon red chili flakes
- One-inch galangal
- Two-bay leaves
- Three-cups water
- 3/4 – cup coconut milk

Instructions:

- Wash and clean the chicken then cuts into cubes.
- Place chicken in an Instant Pot then sprinkles minced garlic, sliced shallot, galangal, green chili flakes, red chili flakes, and bay leaves over the chicken.
- Pour water and coconut milk over the chicken then covers the Instant Pot with the lid and seal it properly.
- Select the *manual* menu then cooks on high for 10 minutes.
- Once it is done, quick release the Instant pot then opens the lid.
- Transfer to a serving dish.

!

Nutrition Info Per Serving:

- Calories: 242
- Total Fat: 13.6g
- Saturated Fat: 9.5g
- Trans Fat: 0g
- Cholesterol: 73mg
- Sodium: 71mg
- Potassium: 580mg
- Total Carb: 4.5g
- Dietary Fiber: 1.2g
- Sugars: 1.8g
- Protein: 25.4g

Serving: 4

Ingredients:

- 1 – pound organic boneless chicken breast
- Two-tablespoons chopped onion
- 4 – whole shallots
- Half-teaspoon pepper
- 1/4 – teaspoon nutmeg
- One-teaspoon paprika
- Two-kaffir lime leaves
- 1/4 – Cup mashed tomato
- 1/4 – Cup unsweetened tomato juice
- One-cup water

Instructions:

- Place all of the ingredients into an Instant Pot then covers it with the lid and seals it properly.
- Select the *manual* menu then cook on high for 10 minutes.
- Once it is done, quick release the Instant pot then open the lid.
- Transfer the chicken together with the gravy to a soup bowl then serves.

!

Nutrition Info Per Serving:

- Calories: 132
- Total Fat: 1.2g
- Saturated Fat: 0.1g
- Trans Fat: 0g
- Cholesterol: 76mg
- Sodium: 135mg
- Potassium: 76mg
- Total Carb: 4.8g
- Dietary Fiber: 0.6g
- Sugars: 1g
- Protein: 26.9g

Serving: 4

Ingredients:

- 1 – pound organic chicken wings
- Two-teaspoons black pepper
- Two-tablespoons lemon juice
- Two-tablespoons avocado oil
- Two-tablespoons low sodium soy sauce
- One-Cup water

Instructions:

- Pour water into an Instant Pot then place a trivet in it.
- Rub the chicken with lemon and black pepper then places the chicken on the prepared trivet.
- Cover the Instant Pot with the lid and seal it properly.
- Select the *manual* menu then cook on high for 10 minutes.
- Once the chicken is done, quick release the Instant pot then open the lid.
- Preheat a saucepan over medium heat then pours avocado oil into it.
- Transfer the cooked chicken to the saucepan then sauté until crisp.
- Drizzle soy sauce over the chicken then stir well.
- Transfer to a serving dish.

!

Nutrition Info Per Serving:

- Calories: 234
- Total Fat: 9.4g
- Saturated Fat: 2.6g
- Trans Fat: 0g
- Cholesterol: 101mg
- Sodium: 402mg
- Potassium: 337mg
- Total Carb: 2g
- Dietary Fiber: 0.7g
- Sugars: 0.3g
- Protein: 33.5g

Serving: 4

Ingredients:

- 1 – pound ground chicken
- Half-Cup almond flour
- Two-organic eggs
- One-teaspoon minced garlic
- One-teaspoon avocado oil
- One-tablespoons sliced shallots
- Half-teaspoon turmeric
- One-inch galangal
- Two-bay leaves
- One-Cup water
- Half-Cup coconut milk

Instructions:

- Combine ground chicken with almond flour, eggs, and minced garlic in a bowl.
- Using your hand, mix the ingredients then shape into medium ball forms. Set aside.
- Select the *sauté* setting in an Instant Pot then pours avocado oil into it.
- Stir in sliced shallots into the pot then sauté until aromatic. Press the cancel button.
- Add turmeric, galangal, and bay leaves into the pot then pours water and coconut milk into the pot. Stir until incorporated.
- Slowly put the balls in the Instant Pot then covers seals it properly.
- Select the *manual* menu then cook on high for 10 minutes.
- Once it is done, quick release the Instant pot then open the lid.
- Transfer to a serving dish then serves.

Nutrition Info Per Serving:

- Calories: 309
- Total Fat: 22.3g
- Saturated Fat: 9.9g
- Trans Fat: 0.1g
- Cholesterol: 179mg
- Sodium: 106mg
- Potassium: 726mg
- Total Carb: 4.6g
- Dietary Fiber: 1.6g
- Sugars: 1.5g
- Protein: 24.9g

Serving: 4

Ingredients:

- 1 – pound chicken thighs
- 1/4 – Cup chopped onion
- One-teaspoon pepper
- One-teaspoon avocado oil
- Two-tablespoons red chili flakes
- Two-tablespoons low sodium soy sauce
- One-Cup water
- 1/4 – Cup mushroom, cut into sticks
- 1/4 – Cup chopped kale

Instructions:

- Select the *sauté* setting in an Instant Pot then pours avocado oil into it.
- Stir in the chopped onion and red chili flakes into the pot then sauté until aromatic. Press the cancel button.
- Add the chicken into the Instant Pot then seasons with pepper.
- Drizzle soy sauce over the chicken then add mushroom sticks into the pot.
- Pour water over the chicken then covers the Instant Pot with the lid and seal it properly.
- Select the *manual* menu then cook on high for 20 minutes.
- Once it is done, quick release the Instant pot then open the lid.
- Add chopped kale into the pot stirs until the kale is wilted.
- Transfer to a serving dish then serve.

!

Nutrition Info Per Serving:

- Calories: 231
- Total Fat: 8.6g
- Saturated Fat: 2.4g
- Trans Fat: 0g
- Cholesterol: 101mg
- Sodium: 402mg
- Potassium: 363mg
- Total Carb: 2.8g
- Dietary Fiber: 0.6g
- Sugars: 0.8g
- Protein: 33.8g

Serving: 4

Ingredients:

- 1 – pound organic chicken breast
- Two-teaspoons minced garlic
- Half-teaspoon paprika
- Half-teaspoon black pepper
- One-tablespoon avocado oil
- 1/4 – Cup water
- 1/4 – Cup chopped lettuce
- Two-tablespoons diced tomato
- Three-tablespoons mayonnaise

Instructions:

- Chop the chicken into chunks then sets aside.
- Select the *Sauté* mode on an Instant Pot then pours avocado oil into the pot.
- Stir in the chicken together with minced garlic, paprika, and black pepper then sautés until aromatic.
- Pour water into the pot then covers the Instant Pot with the lid and seals it properly.
- Select the *manual* menu then cooks on high for 10 minutes.
- Once it is done, quick release the Instant pot then opens the lid.
- Transfer the chicken to a salad dish then add chopped lettuce and tomatoes beside the chicken.
- Drizzle mayonnaise on top then serve.

!

Nutrition Info Per Serving:

- Calories: 207
- Total Fat: 10.1g
- Saturated Fat: 1.1g
- Trans Fat: 0g
- Cholesterol: 75mg
- Sodium: 137mg
- Potassium: 454mg
- Total Carb: 3.7g
- Dietary Fiber: 0.3g
- Sugars: 0.9g
- Protein: 24.4g

Serving: 6

Ingredients:

- 1 – pound fresh prawn
- Two-tablespoons chopped onion
- One-tablespoon chopped celery

For The Sauce:

- Half-Cup tomato puree
- Two-teaspoons minced garlic
- Two-teaspoons sliced shallot
- Three-teaspoons garam masala
- One-teaspoon paprika
- 1/4 – teaspoon turmeric
- One-teaspoon cayenne
- One-tablespoon red chili flakes

Instructions:

- Peel the fresh prawn then sets aside.
- Place all of the sauce ingredients in a food processor then process until smooth.
- Place the peeled prawn in an Instant Pot then add chopped onion into it.
- Pour the sauce mixture over the prawn then mix well.
- Cover the Instant Pot with the lid and seal it properly.
- Select the *manual* menu then cook on high for 3 minutes.
- Once it is done, quick release the Instant pot then open the lid.
- Sprinkle chopped celery over the prawn then stirs well.
- Transfer to a serving dish.

Nutrition Info Per Serving:

- Calories: 104
- Total Fat: 1.4g
- Saturated Fat: 0.4g
- Trans Fat: 0g
- Cholesterol: 159mg
- Sodium: 194mg
- Total Carb: 4.4g
- Dietary Fiber: 0.8g
- Sugars: 1.3g
- Protein: 17.9g

Serving: 4

Ingredients:

- 4 – pounds clams with the shells
- One-teaspoon paprika
- One-tablespoon red chili flakes
- One-tablespoon green chili flakes
- 1/4 – teaspoon black pepper
- One-teaspoon minced garlic
- One-teaspoon turmeric
- Half-Cup water
- 1/4 – Cup coconut milk

Instructions:

- Prepare an oven-safe dish and coat with cooking spray.
- Pour water and coconut milk into the dish then seasons with minced garlic, black pepper, paprika, turmeric, red chili flakes, and green chili flakes.
- Add the clams into the dish then stir until just combined.
- Pour water into the Instant Pot and place a trivet in it.
- Place the dish on the trivet then covers and seals it properly.
- Select the *Manual* setting then cooks for 3 minutes.
- When the Instant Pot beeps, naturally release it and open the lid.
- Transfer the cooked clams to a serving dish together with the gravy.

Nutrition Info Per Serving:

- Calories: 92
- Total Fat: 4.4g
- Saturated Fat: 3.3g
- Trans Fat: 0g
- Cholesterol: 23mg
- Sodium: 57mg
- Potassium: 292mg
- Total Carb: 4g
- Dietary Fiber: 0.7g
- Sugars: 0.8g
- Protein: 9.2g

Serving: 4

Ingredients:

- 1 – pound fresh prawn
- Three-cloves garlic
- 5 – shallots
- One-teaspoon turmeric
- Half-teaspoon pepper
- One-teaspoon avocado oil
- One-inch galangal
- Two-bay leaves
- One-Cup water
- Half-Cup coconut milk
- Two-tablespoons chopped leek

Instructions:

- Wash and clean the prawn then carefully peels them. Set aside.
- Place garlic, shallots, turmeric, and pepper in a food processor. Process until smooth.
- Select the *sauté* setting in an Instant Pot then pours avocado oil into it.
- Stir in the spices mixture into the pot then sauté until aromatic. Press the cancel button.
- Add the prawn into the Instant Pot then seasons with galangal and bay leaves.
- Pour water and coconut milk over the prawn then covers the Instant Pot with the lid and seal it properly.
- Select the *manual* menu then cook on high for 2 minutes.
- Once it is done, quick release the Instant pot then open the lid.
- Transfer to a serving dish then sprinkles chopped leek on top.
- Serve immediately.

Nutrition Info Per Serving:

- Calories: 225
- Total Fat: 9.4g
- Saturated Fat: 7g
- Trans Fat: 0g
- Cholesterol: 239mg
- Sodium: 286mg
- Total Carb: 7.8g
- Dietary Fiber: 1.1g
- Sugars: 1.2g
- Protein: 27.1g

Serving: 4

Ingredients:

- Two-pounds fresh fish
- Two-teaspoons minced garlic
- Two-tablespoons chopped cilantro
- One-tablespoon chopped green chili
- Two-tablespoons fish sauce
- Half-teaspoon black pepper
- Two-tablespoons water

Instructions:

- Prepare an oven-safe dish and coat with cooking spray.
- Place the fish in the dish then seasons with minced garlic, chopped cilantro, green chili, fish sauce, black pepper, water, and lemon juice.
- Pour water into the Instant Pot and place a trivet in it.
- Place the dish on the trivet then covers and seals it properly.
- Select the *Manual* setting then cooks for 3 minutes.
- When the Instant Pot beeps, naturally release it and open the lid.
- Transfer the fish to a serving dish together with the gravy.

Nutrition Info Per Serving:

- Calories: 259
- Total Fat: 5.6g
- Saturated Fat: 0.1g
- Trans Fat: 0g
- Cholesterol: 0mg
- Sodium: 712mg
- Potassium: 47mg
- Total Carb: 1.9g
- Dietary Fiber: 0.1g
- Sugars: 0.6g
- Protein: 50.4g

Serving: 4

Ingredients:

- 1 – pound fresh oyster
- One-tablespoon minced garlic
- 1/4 – teaspoon pepper
- Two-red tomatoes
- One-lemon

Instructions:

- Pour water into the Instant Pot then place a trivet in it.
- Cut the lemon into wedges then sprinkle on the trivet.
- Discard one shell of the oysters then wash and clean them.
- Cut the tomatoes into very small cubes then mix with garlic and pepper.
- Top each oyster with tomato mixture then arranges them on the trivet between the lemon wedges.
- Cover the Instant Pot with the lid then seals it properly.
- Select the *Manual* setting then cooks on high for 3 minutes.
- Once the oysters are done, quick release the Instant Pot then opens the lid.
- Take the oysters out from the Instant Pot then arrange on a serving dish.

!

Nutrition Info Per Serving:

- Calories: 35
- Total Fat: 0.9g
- Saturated Fat: 0.2g
- Trans Fat: 0g
- Cholesterol: 17mg
- Sodium: 38mg
- Potassium: 198mg
- Total Carb: 4.6g
- Dietary Fiber: 1g
- Sugars: 1.8g
- Protein: 3g

Serving: 4

Ingredients:

- 1 – pound salmon fillet
- 1/4 – Cup soy sauce
- One-teaspoon ginger
- One-teaspoon minced garlic
- Two-tablespoons fish sauce
- One-tablespoon lemon juice

Instructions:

- Combine soy sauce with ginger, minced garlic, and fish sauce then mixes well.
- Rub the salmon fillet with the spices mixture then marinates for about 20 minutes. Chill in the refrigerator to keep it fresh.
- Meanwhile, pour water into an Instant Pot then place a trivet in it.
- After 20 minutes, transfer the seasoned fish to the trivet then covers the Instant Pot and seals it properly.
- Select the *manual* setting then cooks on high for 2 minutes.
- Once the pork is done, quick release the Instant Pot then opens the lid.
- Transfer to a serving dish then splash lemon juice over the steamed salmon.

!

Nutrition Info Per Serving:

- Calories: 165
- Total Fat: 7.1g
- Saturated Fat: 1g
- Trans Fat: 0g
- Cholesterol: 50mg
- Sodium: 1644mg
- Potassium: 510mg
- Total Carb: 2.2g
- Dietary Fiber: 0.2g
- Sugars: 0.7g
- Protein: 23.6g

Serving: 4

Ingredients:

- 3 – pounds crab legs
- One-Cup water
- 1/4 – Cup butter, melted
- Two-tablespoons lemon juice

Instructions:

- Pour water in an Instant Pot then place a trivet n it.
- Arrange the crab legs on the trivet then covers the Instant Pot with the lid and seals it properly.
- Select the *Manual* menu then cook on high for 2 minutes.
- Once it is done, quick release the Instant pot then open the lid.
- Take cooked crab legs out from the Instant Pot then place in a bowl.
- Add melted butter into the crabs then splash lemon juice on top. Stir until the crabs are completely coated with butter and lemon.
- Serve immediately.

!

Nutrition Info Per Serving:

- Calories: 164
- Total Fat: 12g
- Saturated Fat: 7.4g
- Trans Fat: 0g
- Cholesterol: 31mg
- Protein: 0.2g
- Sodium: 790mg
- Potassium: 13mg
- Total Carb: 0.2g
- Dietary Fiber: 0g
- Sugars: 0.2g

Serving: 4

Ingredients:

- 1 – pound fresh squids
- Two-teaspoons minced garlic
- Two-teaspoons sliced shallots
- One-tablespoon green chili flakes
- One-tablespoons red chili flakes
- One-teaspoon paprika
- One-teaspoon cayenne
- 5 – kaffir lime leaves
- One-teaspoon soy sauce
- Half-Cup water

Instructions:

- Wash and clean the squids then discard the ink.
- Cut the squids into thick slices then place in an Instant Pot.
- Add the remaining ingredients into the pot then cover the Instant Pot with the lid and seal it properly.
- Select the *manual* menu then cook on high for 20 minutes.
- Once it is done, quick release the Instant pot then open the lid.
- Transfer to a serving dish.

Nutrition Info Per Serving:

- Calories: 126
- Total Fat: 1.7g
- Saturated Fat: 0.4g
- Trans Fat: 0g
- Cholesterol: 264mg
- Sodium: 160mg
- Potassium: 322mg
- Total Carb: 9.1g
- Dietary Fiber: 0.4g
- Sugars: 0.4g
- Protein: 18.1g

Serving: 4

Ingredients:

- Two-pounds fresh crabs
- Two-tablespoons minced garlic
- Half-teaspoon pepper
- One-teaspoon avocado oil
- One-tablespoon oyster sauce
- One-Cup water
- Two-tablespoons chopped leek

Instructions:

- Wash and clean the crabs. Using a brush if it is necessary.
- Once the crabs are clean then cut each crab into halves.
- Select the *Sauté* setting in an Instant Pot then pours avocado oil into it.
- Stir in the minced garlic into the pot then sauté until aromatic. Press the cancel button.
- Add the crabs into the Instant Pot then seasons with pepper.
- Pour water over the crabs then covers the Instant Pot with the lid and seals it properly.
- Select the *Manual* menu then cook on high for 4 minutes.
- Once it is done, quick release the Instant pot then open the lid.
- Sprinkle chopped leek over the crabs then stir well.
- Transfer to a serving dish.

!

Nutrition Info Per Serving:

- Calories: 242
- Total Fat: 4.2g
- Saturated Fat: 0.6g
- Trans Fat: 0g
- Cholesterol: 227mg
- Sodium: 663mg
- Potassium: 765mg
- Total Carb: 2.1g
- Dietary Fiber: 0.3g
- Sugars: 0.2g
- Protein: 46.2g

Serving: 4

Ingredients:

- 1 – pound fresh prawn
- Two-teaspoons sliced garlic
- Half-teaspoon nutmeg
- One-tablespoon red chili flakes
- Half-teaspoon pepper
- 1 and ½ – cups water
- 1/4 – Cup unsweetened tomato juice
- Two-tablespoons tomato paste
- Any kinds of green, as you desired

Instructions:

- Wash and clean the prawn. Peel the prawn then cut the prawn lengthwise.
- Place prawn in an Instant Pot then add greens over the prawn.
- Sprinkle sliced garlic, nutmeg, red chili flakes, and pepper over the prawn then mixes well.
- Pour water, tomato juice, and tomato paste over the prawn then covers the Instant Pot with the lid and seal it properly.
- Select the *manual* menu then cook on high for 4 minutes.
- Once it is done, quick release the Instant pot then open the lid.
- Transfer to a serving dish then sprinkles black pepper on top.
- Garnish with any kinds of green, as you desired. Enjoy warm!

Nutrition Info Per Serving:

- Calories: 160
- Total Fat: 2.2g
- Saturated Fat: 0.7g
- Trans Fat: 0g
- Cholesterol: 239mg
- Sodium: 289mg
- Potassium: 372mg
- Total Carb: 7.3g
- Dietary Fiber: 1.6g
- Sugars: 2.2g
- Protein: 27.1g

Serving: 4

Ingredients:

- 1 – pound fresh shrimps
- Two-teaspoons minced garlic
- Half-teaspoon pepper
- Two-tablespoons lemon juice
- One-cup chopped lettuce
- 1/4 – Cup chopped tomato

Instructions:

- Prepare an oven-safe dish and coat with cooking spray.
- Peel the shrimps then place them in the prepared dish.
- Season the shrimps with minced garlic, pepper, and lemon juice. Using your hand, rub the shrimps until completely seasoned.
- Pour water into the Instant Pot then place a trivet in it.
- Place the dish on the trivet then covers and seals it properly.
- Select the *Manual* setting then cooks for 2 minutes.
- Once the shrimps are done, naturally release it and open the lid.
- Place chopped lettuce and chopped tomato on a serving dish then place the cooked shrimps after the vegetables.

!

Nutrition Info Per Serving:

- Calories: 143
- Total Fat: 2.1g
- Saturated Fat: 0.7g
- Trans Fat: 0g
- Cholesterol: 239mg
- Sodium: 280mg
- Potassium: 257mg
- Total Carb: 3.4g
- Dietary Fiber: 0.4g
- Sugars: 0.6g
- Protein: 26.2g

Serving: 4

Ingredients:

- 1 – pound fresh calamari
- Two-teaspoons minced garlic
- Two-tablespoons sliced shallots
- One-teaspoon black pepper
- One-teaspoon avocado oil
- Half-Cup water
- 1/4 – Cup coconut milk

Instructions:

- Wash and clean the calamari then discards the ink.
- Select *Sauté* menu in an Instant Pot then pour avocado oil into it.
- Once it is hot, stir in minced garlic and sliced shallots into the pot then sautés until wilted and aromatic. Press the *Cancel* button.
- Add calamari into the pot then seasons with black pepper.
- Pour water and coconut milk over the calamari then covers the Instant Pot with the lid and seal it properly.
- Select the *manual* menu then cooks on high for 5 minutes.
- Once it is done, quick release the Instant pot then opens the lid.
- Transfer to a serving dish together with the liquid then Serve warm.

Nutrition Info Per Serving:

- Calories: 98
- Total Fat: 4.8g
- Saturated Fat: 3.2g
- Trans Fat: 0g
- Cholesterol: 130mg
- Sodium: 29mg
- Potassium: 72mg
- Total Carb: 4g
- Dietary Fiber: 0.6g
- Sugars: 0.5g
- Protein: 9.1g

Serving: 4

Ingredients:

- 1 – pound fish fillet
- Two-tablespoons chopped onion
- One-tablespoon chopped lemon grass
- Half-teaspoon ginger
- Half-teaspoon pepper
- 1/4 – teaspoon nutmeg
- One-kaffir lime leaf
- Two-tablespoons mashed tomato
- 1/4 – Cup unsweetened tomato juice
- One-Cup water

Instructions:

- Place fish fillet in an Instant Pot.
- Add the remaining ingredients into the pot then cover it properly.
- Select the *manual* menu then cook on high for 3 minutes.
- Once it is done, quick release the Instant pot then open the lid.
- Transfer the fish together with the gravy to a soup bowl then serves.

Nutrition Info Per Serving:

- Calories: 80
- Total Fat: 3.7g
- Saturated Fat: 1g
- Trans Fat: 0g
- Cholesterol: 10mg
- Sodium: 154mg
- Potassium: 17mg
- Total Carb: 7.6g
- Dietary Fiber: 0.4g
- Sugars: 0.5g
- Protein: 4.2g

Serving: 4

Ingredients:

- 1 – pound fresh fish
- One-tablespoon lemon juice
- One-teaspoon avocado oil
- Four-shallots
- 5 – cloves garlic
- One-teaspoon turmeric
- One-teaspoon ginger
- Two-candlenuts
- One-inch galangal
- One-bay leaf
- 1/4 – Cup cayenne pepper
- Two-lemon grasses
- One-kaffir lime leaf
- Two-tablespoons red chili flakes
- Two-tablespoons green chili flakes
- 1/4 – Cup hot water

Instructions:

- Rub the chicken with lemon juice then let it sit for about 10 minutes.
- Meanwhile, place shallots, garlic, turmeric, ginger, candlenuts, and cayenne pepper in a food processor. Process until smooth then sets aside.
- After 10 minutes, select the *sauté* setting in an Instant Pot then pours avocado oil into it.
- Stir in the spices mixture, galangal, bay leaf, lemon grass, red chili flakes, green chili flakes, and kaffir lime leaf then sautés until aromatic.
- Place the fish in the Instant Pot then mixes with the spices until the fish is completely seasoned. Press the *Cancel* button.
- Pour water over the fish then covers the Instant Pot with the lid and seal it properly.
- Select the *manual* menu then cook on high for 5 minutes.
- Once it is done, naturally release the Instant pot then open the lid.
- Transfer to a serving dish then serves immediately.

Nutrition Info Per Serving:

- Calories: 86
- Total Fat: 3.3g

- Saturated Fat: 0.3g
- Trans Fat: 0g
- Cholesterol: 18mg
- Sodium: 26mg
- Potassium: 291mg
- Total Carb: 6.9g
- Dietary Fiber: 1.2g
- Sugars: 0.9g
- Protein: 7.7g

Classic Salmon Steak

Serving: 4

Ingredients:

- 1 – pound salmon fillet
- Half-teaspoon nutmeg
- Half-teaspoon pepper
- One-tablespoon sesame oil
- Two-tablespoons low sodium soy sauce
- Half-teaspoon cumin
- 1/4 – Cup water
- One-tablespoon chopped celeries
- Half-tablespoon sesame seeds

Instructions:

- Combine nutmeg and pepper in a bowl then mixes well.
- Rub the salmon fillet with the spices mixture then marinates for at 10 minutes.
- Pour water into the Instant Pot then add sesame oil, cumin, and soy sauce. Mix until incorporated.
- Add the salmon fillet into the Instant Pot then covers the Instant Pot with the lid and seals it properly.
- Select the *manual* menu then cooks on high for 3 minutes.
- Once it is done, quick release the Instant pot then opens the lid.
- Transfer the cooked salmon to a plate together with the liquid.
- Sprinkle sesame seeds and chopped celeries over the salmon then serve.

Nutrition Info Per Serving:

- Calories: 195
- Total Fat: 11.1g
- Saturated Fat: 1.6g
- Trans Fat: 0g

- Cholesterol: 50mg
- Sodium: 353mg
- Total Carb: 1.5g
- Dietary Fiber: 0.4g
- Sugars: 0.3g
- Protein: 22.8g

Keto Tuna Casserole

Serving: 4

Ingredients:

- Two-pounds tuna chunks
- One-teaspoon paprika
- Two-organic eggs
- 1/4 – teaspoon pepper
- Half-teaspoon nutmeg
- 1/4 – Cup chopped leek
- Half-Cup avocado wedges

Instructions:

- Prepare an oven-safe dish and coat with cooking spray.
- Pour beef broth and coconut milk into the dish then seasons with minced garlic and pepper. Set aside.
- Place the ground beef in a food processor together with collard green, paprika, chili, almond flour, and eggs. Process until smooth.
- Shape the mixture into ball forms then arrange them in the prepared dish.
- Pour water into the Instant Pot and place a trivet in it.
- Place the dish on the trivet then covers and seals it properly.
- Select the *Manual* setting then cooks for 20 minutes.
- When the Instant Pot beeps, naturally release it and open the lid.
- Transfer the meatballs to a serving dish together with the gravy.
- Sprinkle chopped leek and red chili flakes then serves immediately.

Nutrition Info Per Serving:

- Calories: 111
- Total Fat: 4g
- Saturated Fat: 0.9g
- Trans Fat: 0g
- Cholesterol: 112mg
- Sodium: 283mg
- Total Carb: 2.1g
- Dietary Fiber: 0.9g
- Sugars: 0.5g
- Protein: 16.1g

Serving: 4

Ingredients:

- 1 – pound tuna fillet
- Half-teaspoon black pepper
- Two-tablespoons avocado oil
- Two-tablespoons lemon juice
- Half-teaspoon lemon zest
- 1/4 – teaspoon nutmeg

Instructions:

- Select the *Sauté* setting in an Instant Pot then add the tuna fillet in it.
- Brown each side of the tuna fillet then presses the cancel button.
- Place black pepper, nutmeg, lemon zest, lemon juice, and avocado oil in a bowl then mix well.
- Drizzle the mixture over the tuna fillet then covers the Instant Pot and seals it properly.
- Select the *manual* setting then cooks on high for 3 minutes.
- Once it is done, quick release the Instant Pot then opens the lid.
- Transfer to a serving dish then serves immediately.

Nutrition Info Per Serving:

- Calories: 158
- Total Fat: 4.4g
- Saturated Fat: 1.2g
- Trans Fat: 0g
- Cholesterol: 48mg
- Sodium: 429mg
- Potassium: 305mg
- Total Carb: 0.8g
- Dietary Fiber: 0.5g
- Sugars: 0.2g
- Protein: 27g

Serving: 4

Ingredients:

- 1 – pound fresh squids
- Two-tablespoons chopped onion
- One-teaspoon avocado oil
- 1/4 – Cup diced tomato
- One-cup unsweetened tomato juice
- Half-teaspoon pepper
- One-tablespoon sesame seeds

Instructions:

- Wash and clean the squids then discard the ink.
- Cut the squids into thick slices then set aside.
- Select the *sauté* setting in an Instant Pot then pours avocado oil into it.
- Stir in the chopped onion into the pot then sauté until aromatic. Press the cancel button.
- Add the squids into the Instant Pot together then pour unsweetened tomato juice diced tomato over the squids.
- Season with pepper then cover the Instant Pot with the lid and seal it properly.
- Select the *manual* menu then cook on high for 20 minutes.
- Once it is done, quick release the Instant pot then open the lid.
- Transfer to a serving dish then sprinkle sesame seeds on top.

Nutrition Info Per Serving:

- Calories: 134
- Total Fat: 2.9g
- Saturated Fat: 0.6g
- Trans Fat: 0g
- Cholesterol: 264mg
- Sodium: 57mg
- Potassium: 470mg
- Total Carb: 7.8g
- Dietary Fiber: 0.9g
- Sugars: 2.7g
- Protein: 18.7g

Serving: 4

Ingredients:

- 1 – pound salmon fillet
- 1 and ½ – cups water
- One-teaspoon black pepper
- One-tablespoon lemon juice
- Two-teaspoons minced garlic
- Half-teaspoon paprika

Instructions:

- Place salmon fillet in the Instant Pot then sprinkles black pepper, minced garlic, and paprika on top.
- Splash lemon juice over the salmon then pours water into the Instant Pot.
- Cover the Instant Pot with the lid and seal it properly.
- Select the *Manual* menu then cook on high for 3 minutes.
- Once it is done, quick release the Instant pot then open the lid.
- Transfer to a serving dish together with the gravy then serves immediately.

!

Nutrition Info Per Serving:

- Calories: 84
- Total Fat: 2.9g
- Saturated Fat: 0.5g
- Trans Fat: 0g
- Cholesterol: 21mg
- Sodium: 218mg
- Potassium: 286mg
- Total Carb: 4.8g
- Dietary Fiber: 0.4g
- Sugars: 0.3g
- Protein: 9.3g

Serving: 4

Ingredients:

- 1 – pound fresh prawn
- Two-teaspoons minced garlic
- Two-tablespoons sliced shallots
- One-tablespoon red chili flakes
- 1/4 – teaspoon turmeric
- One-inch galangal
- Two-bay leaves
- Half-teaspoon black pepper
- One-Cup water
- 1/4 – Cup coconut milk

Instructions:

- Wash and clean the prawn. You don't need to peel them.
- Place prawn in an Instant Pot then sprinkles minced garlic, sliced shallot, galangal, red chili flakes, and bay leaves over the prawn.
- Pour water and coconut milk over the prawn then covers the Instant Pot with the lid and seal it properly.
- Select the *manual* menu then cook on high for 4 minutes.
- Once it is done, quick release the Instant pot then open the lid.
- Transfer to a serving dish then sprinkles black pepper on top.
- Garnish with any kinds of green, as you desired. Enjoy warm!

!

Nutrition Info Per Serving:

- Calories: 178
- Total Fat: 5.6g
- Saturated Fat: 3.8g
- Trans Fat: 0g
- Cholesterol: 239mg
- Sodium: 282mg
- Potassium: 272mg
- Total Carb: 4.6g
- Dietary Fiber: 0.6g
- Sugars: 0.6g
- Protein: 26.5g

Serving: 4

Ingredients:

- Two-pounds fresh clams with the shells
- Two-teaspoons minced garlic
- One-teaspoon sliced shallots
- 5 – lemon grasses
- Half-teaspoon pepper
- One-teaspoon avocado oil
- Two-cups water
- Two-tablespoons chopped leek

Instructions:

- Cut the lemon grasses into slices then sets aside.
- Select the *Sauté* setting in an Instant Pot then pours avocado oil into it.
- Stir in the minced garlic, sliced shallots, and sliced lemon grasses then sauté until aromatic. Press the cancel button.
- Add the clams into the Instant Pot then seasons with pepper
- Pour water over the clams then covers the Instant Pot with the lid and seal it properly.
- Select the *Manual* menu then cooks on high for 3 minutes.
- Once it is done, quick release the Instant pot then open the lid.
- Transfer to a serving dish then sprinkles chopped leek on top. Sauté for a few minutes to make the leek wilted.

Nutrition Info Per Serving:

- Calories: 50
- Total Fat: 0.7g
- Saturated Fat: 0.1g
- Trans Fat: 0g
- Cholesterol: 17mg
- Sodium: 34mg
- Total Carb: 4.1g
- Dietary Fiber: 0.2g
- Sugars: 0.1g
- Protein: 6.8g

Serving: 4

Ingredients:

- 1 – pound fresh prawn
- Two-tablespoons minced garlic
- Half-teaspoon pepper
- One-teaspoon avocado oil
- Half-Cup water
- Two-tablespoons chopped celery

Instructions:

- Wash and clean the prawn then sets aside.
- Select the *sauté* setting in an Instant Pot then pours avocado oil into it.
- Stir in the minced garlic into the pot then sauté until aromatic. Press the cancel button.
- Add the prawn into the Instant Pot then seasons with pepper.
- Pour water over the prawn then covers the Instant Pot with the lid and seals it properly.
- Select the *manual* menu then cook on high for 2 minutes.
- Once it is done, quick release the Instant pot then open the lid.
- Transfer to a serving dish then sprinkles chopped celery on top.

Nutrition Info Per Serving:

- Calories: 144
- Total Fat: 2.1g
- Saturated Fat: 0.6g
- Trans Fat: 0g
- Cholesterol: 239mg
- Sodium: 281mg
- Potassium: 226mg
- Total Carb: 3.5g
- Dietary Fiber: 0.3g
- Sugars: 0.1g
- Protein: 26.2g

Serving: 4

Ingredients:

- 3 – pounds mussel
- Two-teaspoons minced garlic
- Two-teaspoons sliced shallots
- One-tablespoon red chili flakes
- One-teaspoon turmeric
- Half-teaspoon curry
- Half-teaspoon pepper
- One-teaspoon avocado oil
- 1 and ½ – cups water
- Two-tablespoons chopped leek

Instructions:

- Discard the shells then wash and clean the mussels.
- Select the *Sauté* setting in an Instant Pot then pours avocado oil into it.
- Stir in the minced garlic, sliced shallots, and red chili flakes into the pot then sauté until aromatic. Press the cancel button.
- Add the mussels into the Instant Pot then season with turmeric, curry, and pepper.
- Pour water over the mussels then covers the Instant Pot with the lid and seal it properly.
- Select the *Manual* menu then cook on high for 2 minutes.
- Once it is done, quick release the Instant pot then open the lid.
- Quickly stir in the chopped leek into the pot then stirs well.
- Transfer to a serving dish then serves immediately.

!

Nutrition Info Per Serving:

- Calories: 84
- Total Fat: 2.9g
- Saturated Fat: 0.5g
- Trans Fat: 0g
- Cholesterol: 21mg
- Sodium: 218mg
- Potassium: 286mg
- Total Carb: 4.8g
- Dietary Fiber: 0.4g
- Sugars: 0.3g
- Protein: 9.3g

Serving: 4

Ingredients:

- 1 – pound fresh squids
- Two-tablespoons minced garlic
- Two-teaspoons coriander
- Three-kaffir lime leaves
- 1/4 – Cup water

Instructions:

- Wash and clean the squids but keep the ink inside.
- Place the squids in an Instant Pot then sprinkles sliced garlic, coriander, and kaffir lime leaves over the squids.
- Pour water into the Instant Pot then covers the Instant Pot with the lid and seal it properly.
- Select the *manual* menu then cook on high for 20 minutes.
- Once it is done, quick release the Instant pot then open the lid.
- Transfer to a serving dish.

Nutrition Info Per Serving:

- Calories: 118
- Total Fat: 1.6g
- Saturated Fat: 0.4g
- Trans Fat: 0g
- Cholesterol: 264mg
- Sodium: 62mg
- Potassium: 297mg
- Total Carb: 7.1g
- Dietary Fiber: 0.1g
- Sugars: 0g
- Protein: 17.9g

Raspberry Dessert

Preparation time: 10 minutes
Cooking time: 2 minutes
Servings: 12

Ingredients:

- ½ cup coconut butter
- ½ cup coconut oil
- ½ cup coconut, unsweetened and shredded
- ½ cup raspberries, dried
- 3 tablespoons stevia

Directions:

1. Set your instant pot on sauté mode, add coconut butter, melt it, add stevia, oil, coconut and raspberries, stir, cover and cook on High for 2 minutes.
2. Spread this on a lined baking sheet, spread well, introduce in the fridge for a couple of hours, slice and serve.

Enjoy!

Nutrition: calories 174, fat 5, fiber 2, carbs 4, protein 7

Preparation time: 10 minutes
Cooking time: 16 minutes
Servings: 8

Ingredients:

- 5 ounces coconut oil, melted
- ½ teaspoon baking powder
- 4 tablespoons stevia
- 1 teaspoon vanilla extract
- 4 ounces cream cheese
- 6 eggs
- ½ cup blueberries
- 1 and ½ cups water

Directions:

1. In a bowl, mix oil with eggs, cream cheese, vanilla, stevia, blueberries and baking powder, blend using an immersion blender and pour into a baking dish.
2. Add the water to your instant pot, add steamer basket, add baking dish inside, cover and cook on High for 16 minutes.
3. Leave aside to cool down, cut into medium bars and serve them cold.

Enjoy!

Nutrition: calories 162, fat 4, fiber 2, carbs 6, protein 8

Preparation time: 50 minutes

Cooking time: 3 minutes

Servings: 2

Ingredients:

- 1 and ½ cups water+ 2 tablespoons water
- 1 tablespoon gelatin
- 2 tablespoons stevia
- 2 tablespoons cocoa powder
- 1 cup coconut milk, hot

Directions:

1. In a bowl, mix milk with stevia and cocoa powder and stir well.
2. In a bowl, mix gelatin with 2 tablespoons water, stir well, add to the cocoa mix, stir and divide into 2 ramekins.
3. Add the water to your instant pot, add the steamer basket, add ramekins inside, cover and cook on High for 3 minutes.
4. Keep puddings in the fridge until you serve.

Nutrition: calories 120, fat 2, fiber 1, carbs 4, protein 3

Preparation time: 10 minutes

Cooking time: 2 minutes

Servings: 4

Ingredients:

- 2 avocados, pitted, peeled and chopped
- 2 teaspoons vanilla extract
- 80 drops stevia
- 1 tablespoon lime juice
- 14 ounces coconut milk

* I and ½ cups water

Directions:

1. In your instant pot, mix avocado with coconut milk, vanilla extract, stevia and lime juice, blend well and divide into 4 ramekins.
2. Add the water to your instant pot, add the steamer basket, add ramekins inside, cover and cook on High for 2 minutes.
3. Keep puddings in the fridge until you serve them.

Nutrition: calories 150, fat 3, fiber 1, carbs 3, protein 4

Peppermint Pudding

Preparation time: 2 hours

Cooking time: 2 minutes

Servings: 3

Ingredients:

* ½ cup coconut oil, melted
* 13 stevia drops
* I tablespoon cocoa powder
* I teaspoon peppermint oil
* 14 ounces canned coconut milk
* I avocado, pitted, peeled and chopped
* 10 drops stevia

Directions:

1. In a bowl, mix coconut oil with cocoa powder and 3 drops stevia, stir well, transfer to a lined container, keep in the fridge for I hour and chop into small pieces.
2. In your instant pot, mix coconut milk with avocado, 10 drops stevia and peppermint oil, blend using an immersion blender, cover pot and cook on High for 2 minutes.
3. Add chocolate chips, stir, divide pudding into bowls and keep in the fridge for I hour before serving.

Nutrition: calories 140, fat 3, fiber 2, carbs 3, protein 4

Preparation time: 10 minutes

Cooking time: 3 minutes

Servings: 4

Ingredients:

- 1 and 2/3 cups coconut milk
- 1 tablespoon gelatin
- 6 tablespoons swerve
- 3 egg yolks
- ½ teaspoon vanilla extract

Directions:

1. In a bowl, mix gelatin with 1 tablespoon coconut milk, stir well and leave aside for now.
2. Set your instant pot on simmer mode, add milk, heat it up, add swerve, egg yolks, vanilla extract and gelatin, stir well, cover pot and cook on High for 2 minutes.
3. Divide everything into 4 ramekins and serve them cold.

Nutrition: calories 140, fat 2, fiber 1, carbs 3, protein 2

Preparation time: 10 minutes

Cooking time: 25 minutes

Servings: 12

Ingredients:

- 6 eggs
- 1 orange, cut into quarters
- 1 and ½ cups water
- 1 teaspoon vanilla extract
- 1 teaspoon baking powder
- 9 ounces almond meal
- 4 tablespoons swerve

- 2 tablespoons orange zest, grated
- 2 ounces stevia
- 4 ounces cream cheese
- 4 ounces coconut yogurt

Directions:

1. In your food processor, mix orange with almond meal, swerve, eggs, baking powder and vanilla extract, pulse well and transfer to a cake pan.
2. Add the water to your instant pot, add steamer basket, add cake pan inside, cover and cook on High for 25 minutes.
3. In a bowl, mix cream cheese with orange zest, coconut yogurt and stevia and stir well.
4. Spread this well over cake, slice and serve it.

Nutrition: calories 170, fat 13, fiber 2, carbs 4, protein 4

Walnuts Cream

Preparation time: 10 minutes

Cooking time: 1 minute

Servings: 6

Ingredients:

- 2 ounces coconut oil
- 4 tablespoons cocoa powder
- 1 teaspoon vanilla extract
- 1 cup walnuts, chopped
- 4 tablespoons stevia

Directions:

1. In your instant pot, mix cocoa powder with oil, vanilla, walnuts and stevia, blend using an immersion blender, cover pot and cook on High for 1 minute.
2. Transfer to a bowl, leave in the fridge for a couple of hours and serve.

Nutrition: calories 100, fat 5, fiber 1, carbs 3, protein 4

Preparation time: 10 minutes

Cooking time: 30 minutes

Servings: 6

Ingredients:

- 1 and 1/3 pint coconut milk
- 1 and ½ cups water
- 4 tablespoons lemon zest
- 4 eggs
- 5 tablespoons swerve
- 2 tablespoons lemon juice

Directions:

1. In a bowl, mix eggs with milk, swerve, lemon zest and lemon juice, whisk well and pour into 6 ramekins.
2. Add the water to your instant pot, add steamer basket, add ramekins, cover pot and cook on High for 20 minutes.
3. Leave cream to cool down before servings.

Nutrition: calories 120, fat 2, fiber 2, carbs 5, protein 3

Preparation time: 1 minute

Cooking time: 3 minutes

Servings: 6

Ingredients:

- ½ cup coconut cream
- 4 ounces dark chocolate, unsweetened and chopped

Directions:

1. In your instant pot, mix cream with dark chocolate, cover pot and cook on High for 3 minutes.
2. Stir your cream really well, divide into dessert cups and serve cold.

Nutrition: calories 78, fat 2, fiber 1, carbs 3, protein 1

Preparation time: 10 minutes

Cooking time: 2 minutes

Servings: 4

Ingredients:

- 3 tablespoons cocoa powder
- 14 ounces coconut cream
- 1 cup blackberries
- 1 cup raspberries
- 2 tablespoons stevia

Directions:

1. In your instant pot, mix cream with cocoa, stevia, blackberries and raspberries, stir, cover and cook on High for 2 minutes.
2. Divide into dessert cups and serve cold.

Nutrition: calories 145, fat 4, fiber 2, carbs 6, protein 2

Preparation time: 10 minutes

Cooking time: 2 minutes

Servings: 4

Ingredients:

- 1 and ¾ cups coconut cream
- 2 teaspoons stevia
- 1 cup strawberries

Directions:

1. In your instant pot, mix cream with stevia and strawberries, stir, cover and cook on High for 2 minutes.
2. Divide into bowls and serve cold.

Nutrition: calories 155, fat 2, fiber 1, carbs 5, protein 4

Preparation time: 10 minutes

Cooking time: 25 minutes

Servings: 2

Ingredients:

- 1 and ½ teaspoons caramel extract
- 1 cup water
- 2 ounces cream cheese
- 2 eggs
- 1 and ½ tablespoons swerve

For the sauce:

- 2 tablespoons swerve
- 2 tablespoons ghee
- ¼ teaspoon caramel extract

Directions:

1. In your blender, mix cream cheese with water, 1 and ½ tablespoons swerve, 1 and ½ teaspoons caramel extract and eggs, pulse well and divide into 2 greased ramekins.
2. Add the water to your instant pot, add steamer basket, add ramekins inside, cover and cook on High for 20 minutes.
3. Meanwhile, put the ghee in a pot, heat up over medium heat, add ¼ teaspoon caramel extract and 2 tablespoons swerve, stir well, cook for a few minutes and pour over caramel pudding.

Enjoy!

Nutrition: calories 174, fat 7, fiber 1, carbs 2, protein 4

Preparation time: 10 minutes

Cooking time: 2 minutes

Servings: 4

Ingredients:

- ½ cup chia seeds
- 2 cups almond milk, unsweetened
- 1 teaspoon vanilla extract
- ¼ cup peanut butter, unsweetened
- 1 teaspoon vanilla stevia

Directions:

1. In your instant pot, mix milk with chia seeds, peanut butter, vanilla extract and stevia, stir, cover and cook on High for 2 minutes
2. Divide into dessert glasses and leave in the fridge for 10 minutes before serving,

Nutrition: calories 120, fat 1, fiber 2, carbs 4, protein 2

Pumpkin Cream

Preparation time: 10 minutes

Cooking time: 5 minutes

Servings: 6

Ingredients:

- 1 tablespoon gelatin
- ¼ cup warm water
- 14 ounces coconut milk
- 14 ounces pumpkin puree
- A pinch of salt
- 2 teaspoons vanilla extract
- 1 teaspoon cinnamon powder
- 1 teaspoon pumpkin pie spice

- 8 scoops stevia
- 3 tablespoons erythritol

Directions:

1. In your instant pot, mix pumpkin puree with coconut milk, a pinch of salt, vanilla extract, cinnamon powder, stevia, erythritol and pumpkin pie spice, stir well, cover and cook on High for 4 minutes.
2. In a bowl, mix gelatin and water and stir.
3. Add this over pumpkin cream, stir, divide custard into ramekins and serve them cold.

Nutrition: calories 160, fat 2, fiber 1, carbs 3, protein 4

Chia Jam

Preparation time: 15 minutes

Cooking time: 5 minutes

Servings: 22

Ingredients:

- 3 tablespoons chia seeds
- 2 and ½ cups cherries, pitted
- ½ teaspoon vanilla powder
- Zest from ½ lemon, grated
- ¼ cup erythritol
- 10 drops stevia
- 1 cup water

Directions:

1. In your instant pot, mix cherries with water, stevia, erythritol, vanilla powder, chia seeds and lemon peel, stir, cover and cook on High for 5 minutes.
2. Divide into dessert cups and serve cold.

Nutrition: calories 160, fat 1, fiber 1, carbs 2, protein 0.5

Preparation time: 5 minutes

Cooking time: 10 minutes

Servings: 6

Ingredients:

- Flesh from 1 melon
- 1 ounce stevia
- 1 cup natural apple juice
- 1 tablespoon ghee
- Juice of 1 lemon

Directions:

1. Put melon and apple juice in your instant pot, cover, cook on High for 7 minutes, transfer to a blender, add lemon juice, ghee and stevia, pulse well and return to your instant pot.

2. Set on simmer mode, cook for a couple more minutes, divide into dessert cups and serve.

Nutrition: calories 73, fat 1, fiber 1, carbs 2, protein 2

Peach Cream

Preparation time: 5 minutes

Cooking time: 3 minutes

Servings: 6

Ingredients:

- 10 ounces peaches, stoned and chopped
- A pinch of nutmeg, ground
- 2 tablespoons coconut flakes
- 3 tablespoons stevia
- ½ cup water
- 1/8 teaspoon cinnamon powder
- 1/8 teaspoon almond extract

Directions:

1. In your instant pot, mix peaches with nutmeg, coconut, stevia, almond extract and cinnamon, stir, cover and cook at High for 3 minutes.

2. Divide into small cups and serve.

Nutrition: calories 90, fat 2, fiber 1, carbs 3, protein 5

Preparation time: 10 minutes

Cooking time: 10 minutes

Servings: 6

Ingredients:

- 4 tablespoons stevia
- 3 cups peaches, cored and roughly chopped
- 6 tablespoons natural apple juice
- 2 teaspoons lemon zest, grated

Directions:

1. In your instant pot mix peaches with stevia, apple juice and lemon zest, stir, cover and cook at High for 10 minutes.
2. Divide into small cups and serve cold.

Nutrition: calories 80, fat 2, fiber 2, carbs 5, protein 5

Preparation time: 10 minutes

Cooking time: 20 minutes

Servings: 6

Ingredients:

- 11 ounces stevia
- 11 ounces water
- 1 and ½ pounds chestnuts, halved and peeled

Directions:

1. In your instant pot, mix stevia with water and chestnuts, stir, cover and cook on High for 20 minutes.
2. Blend using your immersion blender, divide into small cups and serve.

Enjoy!

Nutrition: calories 82, fat 1, fiber 0, carbs 5, protein 3

Preparation time: 60 minutes

Cooking time: 50 minutes

Servings: 12

Ingredients:

For the crust:

- 4 tablespoons melted ghee
- 1 and ½ cups chocolate cookie crumbs

For the filling:

- 24 ounces cream cheese, soft
- 2 tablespoons coconut flakes
- 3 tablespoons stevia
- 3 eggs
- 1 tablespoon vanilla extract
- Cooking spray
- 1 cup water
- ½ cup Greek yogurt
- 5 ounces white chocolate, unsweetened and melted
- 5 ounces bittersweet chocolate, melted

Directions:

1. In a bowl mix cookie crumbs with ghee, stir well, press on the bottom of a cake pan that you've greased with cooking spray, and lined with parchment paper.
2. In a bowl, mix cream cheese with coconut, stevia, eggs, vanilla and yogurt, whisk well and leave aside for a few minutes.
3. Put milk chocolate in a heatproof bowl and heat up in the microwave for 30 seconds.
4. Add white and bittersweet chocolate, stir well again and pour over cookie crust.

5. Add the water to your instant pot, add steamer basket, and cake, cover and cook on High for 45 minutes.

6. Slice and serve cold.

Nutrition: calories 267, fat 4, fiber 7, carbs 10, protein 7

Banana Cake

Preparation time: 10 minutes

Cooking time: 30 minutes

Servings: 6

Ingredients:

- 4 tablespoons stevia
- 1/3 cup ghee, soft
- 1 teaspoon vanilla extract
- 1 egg
- 2 bananas, peeled and mashed
- 1 teaspoon baking powder
- 1 and ½ cups coconut flour
- ½ teaspoons baking soda
- 1/3 cup coconut milk
- 1 and ½ teaspoons keto cream of tartar
- 2 cups water
- Olive oil cooking spray

Directions:

1. In a bowl, mix milk with cream of tartar, stevia, ghee, egg, vanilla and bananas and stir everything.

2. Add flour, baking powder and baking soda, stir well and pour into a cake pan that you've greased with cooking spray.

3. Add the water to your instant pot, add steamer basket, and cake pan, cover and cook on High for 30 minutes.

4. Slice and serve cold.

Enjoy!

Nutrition: calories 214, fat 2, fiber 2, carbs 6, protein 8

Preparation time: 10 minutes

Cooking time: 35 minutes

Servings: 12

Ingredients:

- 2 cups coconut flour
- 1 teaspoon baking soda
- ¾ teaspoon pumpkin pie spice
- ¾ cup stevia
- 1 banana, mashed
- ½ teaspoon baking powder
- 2 tablespoons coconut oil
- ½ cup Greek yogurt
- 8 ounces canned pumpkin puree
- Cooking spray
- 1-quart water
- 1 egg
- ½ teaspoon vanilla extract
- 2/3 cup chocolate chips

Directions:

1. In a bowl, mix flour with baking soda, baking powder, pumpkin spice, stevia, oil, banana, yogurt, pumpkin puree, vanilla and egg and stir using a mixer.
2. Add chocolate chips, stir, pour into a cake pan greased with cooking spray and cover with some tin foil.
3. Add the water to your instant pot, add steamer basket, add cake pan inside, cover and cook on High for 35 minutes.
4. Slice cake and serve cold.

Enjoy!

Nutrition: calories 200, fat 3, fiber 3, carbs 6, protein 8

Preparation time: 10 minutes

Cooking time: 1 hour and 10 minutes

Servings: 6

Ingredients:

- 3 cups apples, cored and cubed
- 4 tablespoons stevia
- 1 tablespoon vanilla extract
- 2 eggs
- 1 tablespoon apple pie spice
- 2 cups coconut flour
- 2 tablespoons ghee, melted
- 1 tablespoon baking powder
- 1 cup water

Directions:

1. In a bowl mix egg with ghee, apple pie spice, stevia, apples, flour and baking powder, stir and pour into a cake pan.
2. Add the water to your instant pot, add steamer basket, add cake pan inside, cover and cook on High for 1 hour.
3. Leave the cake to cool down, slice and serve.

Enjoy!

Nutrition: calories 89, fat 1, fiber 2, carbs 5, protein 4

Preparation time: 10 minutes

Cooking time: 25 minutes

Servings: 8

Ingredients:

- 1 apple, sliced
- 1 apple, chopped
- 1 cup ricotta cheese
- 3 tablespoons stevia
- 1 tablespoon lemon juice
- 1 egg
- 1 teaspoon vanilla extract
- 3 tablespoons olive oil
- 1 cup coconut flour
- 2 teaspoons baking powder
- 1/8 teaspoon cinnamon powder
- 1 teaspoon baking soda
- 2 cups water

Directions:

1. In a bowl, mix all apples with lemon juice and half of the stevia, toss and leave aside.
2. Line a cake pan with some parchment paper, grease with some oil, dust with some flour and spread half of the apples.
3. In a bowl, mix the egg with cheese, the rest of the stevia, vanilla extract, oil, flour, baking powder and soda, the rest of the apples and cinnamon and stir.
4. Pour everything into the cake pan and cover with tin foil.
5. Add the water to your instant pot, add steamer basket, and cake pan, cover and cook on High for 25 minutes.
6. Turn cake upside down, slice and serve.

Enjoy!

Nutrition: calories 210, fat 4, fiber 5, carbs 12, protein 5

Preparation time: 10 minutes
Cooking time: 20 minutes
Servings: 4

Ingredients:

- 1/8 teaspoon almond extract
- 2 cups water
- 1 cup coconut flour
- ½ cup cocoa powder
- 4 tablespoons stevia
- 3 tablespoons olive oil
- 3 eggs
- 2 teaspoons baking powder
- ½ cup almonds, sliced

Directions:

1. In a bowl, mix cocoa powder, almond extract, flour, eggs, stevia, oil, baking powder and almonds, whisk well and pour everything into a greased cake pan.
2. Add the water to your instant pot, add steamer basket, and cake pan, cover and cook on High for 20 minutes.
3. Slice and serve cold.

Enjoy!

Nutrition: calories 162, fat 4, fiber 2, carbs 18, protein 3

Preparation time: 1 hour
Cooking time: 15 minutes
Servings: 6

Ingredients:

- 2 cups coconut cream
- 1 teaspoon cinnamon powder
- 6 egg yolks
- 5 tablespoons stevia
- Zest from 1 lemon, grated
- A pinch of nutmeg
- 2 cups water

Directions:

1. Heat up a pan with the coconut cream over medium heat, add cinnamon and orange zest, stir, bring to a simmer, take off heat and leave aside to cool down.
2. Add egg yolks and stevia, stir well, strain and divide this into small ramekins.
3. Add the water to your instant pot, add steamer basket, add ramekins, cover pot and cook on Low for 10 minutes.
4. Sprinkle nutmeg on top and serve cold.

Enjoy!

Nutrition: calories 200, fat 5, fiber 2, carbs 10, protein 13

Preparation time: 10 minutes

Cooking time: 10 minutes

Servings: 4

Ingredients:

- 4 pears
- Juice of 1 lemon
- Zest from 1 lemon, grated
- 26 ounces grape juice
- ½ vanilla bean
- 4 peppercorns
- 2 rosemary sprigs

Directions:

1. In your instant pot, mix grape juice with lemon juice, lemon zest, vanilla, rosemary, peppercorns and pears, cover pot and cook on High for 10 minutes.
2. Divide into bowls and serve.

Nutrition: calories 152, fat 3, fiber 6, carbs 8, protein 12

Preparation time: 30 minutes

Cooking time: 18 minutes

Servings: 6

Ingredients:

- 1 cup cauliflower rice
- ½ cup water
- 3 cups coconut milk
- ½ cup dates, chopped
- 1 cinnamon stick
- 1 cup pumpkin puree
- 4 tablespoons stevia
- 1 teaspoon vanilla extract

Directions:

1. Put cauliflower rice in your instant pot, add water, milk, dates and cinnamon, stir, cover and cook on High for 13 minutes.
2. Add pumpkin puree, stevia and vanilla, stir, set the pot on Simmer mode and cook for 5 minutes.
3. Discard cinnamon, divide pudding into bowls and serve.

Nutrition: calories 120, fat 3, fiber 3, carbs 8, protein 5

Preparation time: 10 minutes

Cooking time: 4 minutes

Servings: 12

Ingredients:

- 8 pears, cored and roughly chopped
- 2 apples, peeled, cored and roughly chopped
- ¼ cup natural apple juice
- 1 teaspoon cinnamon powder

Directions:

1. In your instant pot, mix pears with apples, cinnamon and apple juice, stir, cover, cook on High for 4 minutes, blend with your immersion blender, leave aside to cool down, divide into small dessert cups and serve.

Nutrition: calories 90, fat 0, fiber 2, carbs 19, protein 2

Preparation time: 10 minutes

Cooking time: 10 minutes

Servings: 6

Ingredients:

- 4 and ½ cups peaches, peeled and cubed
- Stevia to the taste
- 1 teaspoon ginger, grated
- 2 cups water

Directions:

1. In your instant pot, mix peaches with stevia, ginger and water, stir, cover and cook on High for 10 minutes.
2. Divide into small cups, cool down and serve.

Enjoy!

Nutrition: calories 82, fat 1, fiber 2, carbs 3, protein 2

Strawberries Compote

Preparation time: 10 minutes

Cooking time: 7 minutes

Servings: 8

Ingredients:

- 1 cup blueberries
- 2 cups strawberries, chopped
- 2 tablespoons lemon juice
- Stevia to the taste
- 1 tablespoon water

Directions:

1. In your instant pot, mix blueberries with strawberries, lemon juice, stevia and water, stir, cover and cook on High for 7 minutes.
2. Divide into cups and serve cold.

Nutrition: calories 200, fat 1, fiber 3, carbs 12, protein 3

Sweet Peaches

Preparation time: 10 minutes

Cooking time: 6 minutes

Servings: 3

Ingredients:

- 6 peaches, insides discarded
- ¼ cup coconut flour
- 2 tablespoons stevia
- 2 tablespoons coconut butter
- ½ teaspoon cinnamon powder
- 1 teaspoon almond extract
- 1 cup water

Directions:

1. In a bowl, mix flour with stevia, butter, cinnamon and almond, stir well and stuff peaches with this mix.
2. Add the water to your instant pot, add steamer basket, add peaches, cover and cook on High for 6 minutes.
3. Divide into cups and serve them cold.

Nutrition: calories 152, fat 2, fiber 2, carbs 9, protein 3

Preparation time: 10 minutes

Cooking time: 4 minutes

Servings: 4

Ingredients:

- 8 peaches, chopped
- Stevia to the taste
- 1 teaspoon cinnamon powder
- 1 teaspoon vanilla extract
- 1 cup water

Directions:

1. In your instant pot, mix peaches with stevia, water, cinnamon and vanilla, stir, cover and cook on High for 4 minutes.
2. Divide into bowls and serve cold.

Nutrition: calories 120, fat 2, fiber 2, carbs 8, protein 2

Apple Cobbler

Preparation time: 10 minutes

Cooking time: 12 minutes

Servings: 4

Ingredients:

- 3 apples, cored and roughly chopped
- 2 pears, cored and roughly chopped
- 1 and ½ cup hot water
- 2 tablespoons coconut flakes
- 3 tablespoon stevia
- 1 teaspoon cinnamon powder

Directions:

1. In your instant pot, mix apples with pears, water, coconut, stevia and cinnamon, stir, cover and cook on High for 12 minutes.
2. Divide into bowls and serve cold.

Enjoy!

Nutrition: calories 162, fat 2, fiber 2, carbs 6, protein 2

Preparation time: 10 minutes
Cooking time: 25 minutes
Servings: 6

Ingredients:

- 1 cup natural applesauce
- 3 eggs, whisked
- 1 tablespoon vanilla extract
- 4 tablespoons stevia
- 2 cups zucchini, grated
- 2 and ½ cups coconut flour
- ½ cup baking cocoa powder
- 1 teaspoon baking soda
- ¼ teaspoon baking powder
- 1 teaspoon cinnamon powder
- ½ cup walnuts, chopped
- 2 cups water

Directions:

1. In a bowl, mix zucchini with stevia, vanilla, eggs, applesauce, flour, cocoa powder, baking soda, baking powder, cinnamon and walnuts, stir and pour into a cake pan.
2. Add the water to your instant pot, add steamer basket, and cake pan, cover and cook on High for 20 minutes.
3. Slice and serve cold.

Enjoy!

Nutrition: calories 192, fat 3, fiber 6, carbs 8, protein 3

Preparation time: 10 minutes

Cooking time: 30 minutes

Servings: 4

Ingredients:

- 1/3 cup water
- 1 pound strawberries, chopped
- 1 pound rhubarb, chopped
- 3 tablespoon stevia
- 1 tablespoon mint, chopped
- 1 pound strawberries, chopped

Directions:

1. In your instant pot, mix water with strawberries, rhubarb and stevia, stir, cover and cook on High for 20 minutes.
2. Add mint, stir, divide into cups and serve cold.

Nutrition: calories 91, fat 1, fiber 1, carbs 8, protein 1

Carrot, Pecans and Raisins Cake

Preparation time: 10 minutes

Cooking time: 1 hour

Servings: 6

Ingredients:

- 1 and ½ cups water
- A drizzle of coconut oil, melted
- 4 tablespoons stevia
- 2 eggs
- ½ cup coconut flour
- ½ teaspoon allspice
- ½ teaspoon cinnamon powder
- A pinch of nutmeg
- ½ teaspoon baking soda
- ½ cup pecans, chopped
- ½ cup carrots, grated
- ½ cup raisins
- 1 cup coconut flakes

For the sauce:

- 4 tablespoons ghee
- Stevia to the taste
- ¼ cup coconut cream

- ¼ teaspoon cinnamon powder

Directions:

1. In a bowl, mix eggs with 4 tablespoons stevia, flour, allspice, cinnamon powder, nutmeg, baking soda, carrots, pecans, raisins and coconut flakes, whisk well and pour into a cake pan greased with some coconut oil.
2. Add the water to your instant pot, add the steamer basket, add cake pan inside, cover and cook on High for 50 minutes.
3. Meanwhile, heat up a pan with the ghee over medium heat, add stevia to the taste, coconut cream and cinnamon powder, stir and cook for 2 minutes.
4. Drizzle this over cake, slice and serve.

Nutrition: calories 271, fat 4, fiber 4, carbs 17, protein 6

Fresh Figs

Preparation time: 10 minutes

Cooking time: 3 minutes

Servings: 4

Ingredients:

- 1 cup natural grape juice
- 1 pound figs
- ½ cup pine nuts, toasted
- 4 tablespoons stevia

Directions:

1. In your instant pot, mix grape juice with figs and stevia, cover pot and cook on High for 3 minutes.
2. Divide this into bowls, sprinkle pine nuts on top and serve.

Enjoy!

Nutrition: calories 100, fat 0, fiber 1, carbs 9, protein 1

Preparation time: 10 minutes

Cooking time: 10 minutes

Servings: 4

Ingredients:

- 1 tablespoon stevia
- 2 cups baby carrots
- 1 tablespoon ghee
- ½ cup water

Directions:

1. In your instant pot, mix carrots with stevia, ghee and water, stir, cover and cook on High for 10 minutes.
2. Divide into dessert cups and serve.

Nutrition: calories 100, fat 1, fiber 1, carbs 2, protein 2

Pear Pudding

Preparation time: 5 minutes

Cooking time: 7 minutes

Servings: 4

Ingredients:

- 1 cup water
- 2 cups pears, chopped
- 2 cups coconut milk
- 1 tablespoon ghee
- 3 tablespoons stevia
- ½ teaspoon cinnamon powder
- 1 cup coconut flakes
- ½ cup walnuts, chopped

Directions:

1. In a pudding pan, mix milk with stevia, ghee, coconut, cinnamon, pears and walnuts and stir.
2. Add the water to your instant pot, add steamer basket, add pudding pan, cover and cook on High for 7 minutes.
3. Divide into bowls and serve.

Nutrition: calories 172, fat 3, fiber 4, carbs 8, protein 7

Preparation time: 10 minutes

Cooking time: 10 minutes

Servings: 4

Ingredients:

- 1 plum, chopped
- 1 and ½ cups water
- 1 pear, chopped
- 1 apple, chopped
- 2 tablespoons stevia
- 3 tablespoons coconut oil
- ½ teaspoon cinnamon powder
- ¼ cup pecans, toasted and chopped
- ¼ cup coconut, shredded

Directions:

1. In a bowl, mix plum with pear, apple, stevia, oil, cinnamon, coconut and pecans, stir and transfer to a round pan.
2. Add water to your instant pot, add steamer basket, add pan inside, cover and cook on High for 10 minutes.
3. Divide into bowls and serve.

Enjoy!

Nutrition: calories 152, fat 2, fiber 2, carbs 8, protein 7

Preparation time: 10 minutes

Cooking time: 13 minutes

Servings: 6

Ingredients:

- 2 cups water
- 1 tablespoon melted ghee
- 1 cup pumpkin puree
- 1 cup coconut flakes
- 3 tablespoons stevia
- 2 teaspoons cinnamon powder
- 1 teaspoon pumpkin pie spice

Directions:

1. Set your instant pot on sauté mode, add ghee, heat it up, add coconut flakes, pumpkin, water, cinnamon, stevia and spice, stir, cover and cook on High for 13 minutes.
2. Divide into bowls and serve.

Nutrition: calories 182, fat 2, fiber 1, carbs 8, protein 4

Carrot and Chia Seed Pudding

Preparation time: 10 minutes

Cooking time: 10 minutes

Servings: 4

Ingredients:

- 1 cup coconut flakes
- 2 cups water
- 1 tablespoon ghee
- 3 tablespoons stevia
- 2 teaspoons cinnamon powder
- 1 cup carrots, grated
- ¼ cup chia seeds

Directions:

1. Select the Sauté mode on your instant pot, add ghee, heat it up, add coconut, water, stevia, cinnamon, carrots and chia seeds, stir, cover and cook on High for 10 minutes.
2. Divide into bowls and serve cold.

Nutrition: calories 132, fat 2, fiber 2, carbs 9, protein 4

Preparation time: 10 minutes
Cooking time: 10 minutes
Servings: 4

Ingredients:

- 1 and ½ cups cauliflower rice
- 1 and ½ teaspoon cinnamon powder
- 4 tablespoons stevia
- 2 tablespoons ghee
- 2 apples, cored and sliced
- 1 cup natural apple juice
- 3 cups coconut milk

Directions:

1. Set your instant pot on Sauté mode, add ghee, heat it up, add cauliflower rice, stevia, apples, apple juice, milk and cinnamon, stir, cover and cook on High for 10 minutes.
2. Divide into bowls and serve warm.

Enjoy!

Nutrition: calories 110, fat 2, fiber 3, carbs 12, protein 4

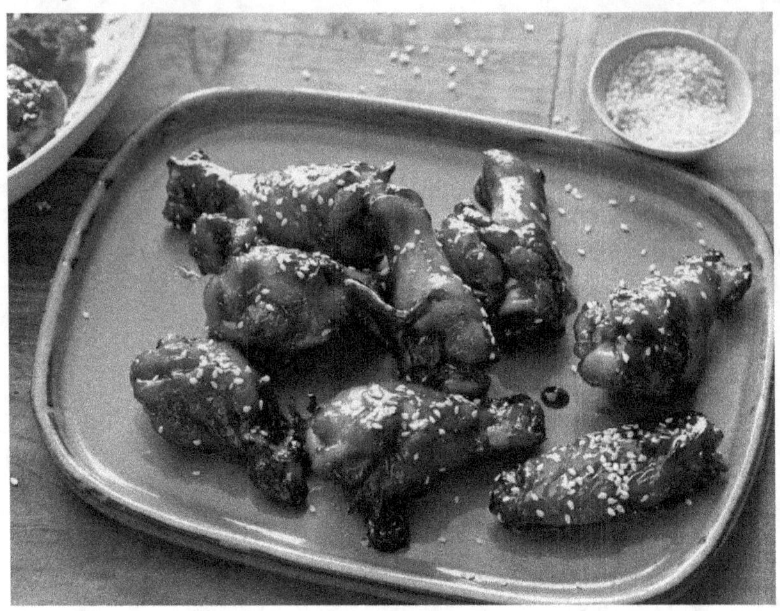

In this special section, we gives you tasty ketogenic recipes that can be put together in express time and cooked using a slow cooker.

These recipes are Keto friendly and help you develop the body of your dreams. The recipes have been designed keeping in mind the needs of health conscious people who wish to develop a lean and healthy body by altering their current diet and include healthier ingredients.

Spicy Chicken Coconut Soup

Serves: 4

Preparation time: 10 minutes

Nutritional values per serving:

Calories - 339, Fat – 25.8 g, Carbohydrates – 11.7 g, Protein – 15.7 g

Ingredients:

- 1 pound chicken breasts, skinless, boneless, cut into 1 inch cubes
- 1 ½ stalks fresh lemongrass, chopped into 2-inch pieces, crushed
- 1 cup mushroom, sliced
- 6 slices ginger (each of about an inch), crushed
- 4 cups chicken broth

- 1 can coconut milk
- 1 ½ tablespoons Vietnamese fish sauce
- 1 ½ tablespoons chili paste
- ¼ teaspoon lime zest, grated
- 2 tablespoons lime juice + extra to serve
- 2 thin lime slices to garnish
- 2 tablespoons fresh cilantro, chopped
- Pepper to taste

Method:

1. Add all the ingredients except cilantro and lemon slices into the slow cooker.
2. Close the lid. Set cooker on 'Low' option and timer for 4-5 hours or on 'High' option and timer for 2-2 ½ hours.
3. Remove the chicken with a slotted spoon and set aside.
4. Let the remaining ingredients in the pot sit for a while. Skim off any fat that is floating on top.
5. Strain the broth through a wire mesh strainer. Press the solid part to get as much juice as possible.
6. Pour the broth back into the slow cooker. Add coconut milk and stir.
7. Add chicken and stir.
8. Cover and cook on 'High' for 30 minutes.
9. Ladle into soup bowls. Garnish with cilantro and lime slices and serve. Drizzle some more lime juice if desired.

Tasty Hot and Sour Shrimp Soup

Serves: 2

Preparation time: 15 minutes

Nutritional values per serving:

Calories - 224, Fat – 8.7 g, Carbohydrates – 7.6 g, Protein – 27.7g

Ingredients:

- 8 to 10 shrimp, peeled, with its tail on, and deveined, set aside the shells
- 1 small onion, chopped
- 1-inch piece galangal, peeled, chopped into thick slices
- 2 fresh kaffir leaves or ¼ teaspoon lemon zest, grated
- 2 ½ cups chicken broth
- ½ small green zucchini, sliced
- 1 tablespoon coconut oil, divided
- 2 cloves garlic
- 1 stalk lemon grass, chopped into 1-inch pieces
- 1 Thai red chili, roughly chopped
- ¼ pound cremini or shiitake or oyster or button mushrooms, rinsed, sliced into wedges
- 1 tablespoon fresh lime juice
- 1 tablespoon fish sauce
- 2 tablespoons fresh basil, chopped
- 2 tablespoons fresh cilantro, chopped
- Salt to taste
- Pepper to taste

Method:

1. Place a skillet over medium heat. Add ½ tablespoon coconut oil. When the oil is heated, add shrimp shells that were kept aside and stir constantly until they turn red in color and lose the ammonia fragrance.
2. Add onions, galangal, garlic, lemon grass, kaffir lime leaves or fresh lime zest, Thai red chili, salt, and pepper. Sauté for a few minutes until the onions turn translucent.
3. Transfer into the slow cooker. Add broth and stir.
4. Close the lid. Set cooker on 'High' option and timer for 30 minutes.
5. Remove the shrimp shells with a slotted spoon. Discard the shells.
6. Transfer the stock back into the slow cooker.

7. Add the remaining coconut oil into the skillet. When the oil is heated, add zucchini slices and mushroom and season with salt and pepper. Sauté until tender.

8. Transfer into the slow cooker. Add shrimp into the pot and stir.

9. Close the lid. Set the cooker on 'High' and timer for 15-20 minutes or until the shrimp turns opaque.

10. Add lime juice, salt, pepper, and fish sauce. Stir well. Taste and adjust the seasoning if necessary.

11. Add fresh cilantro and basil and stir.

12. Ladle into soup bowls and serve immediately.

Turkish Lamb & Veggies Stew

Serves: 2

Preparation time: 15 minutes

Nutritional values per serving:

Calories - 190, Fat – 8 g, Carbohydrates – 20 g, Protein – 16 g

Ingredients:

- 1 large onion, thinly sliced
- 1 medium sweet potato, peeled, cut into thick slices
- 1 small zucchini, cut into thick slices
- 1 small eggplant, cut into thick slices
- ¼ pound green beans, trimmed
- 7 ounces canned diced tomatoes
- ¾ pound lean leg of lamb, boneless, trimmed of fat, chopped into bite size pieces
- 3 bay leaves
- ¼ teaspoon dried oregano
- 1 teaspoon salt, divided
- 2 cloves garlic, minced
- Freshly ground pepper to taste
- 2 teaspoons extra virgin olive oil, divided

Method:

1. Sprinkle salt and pepper over the lamb.
2. Place a heavy skillet over medium heat. Add half the oil. When the oil is heated, add lamb and cook until brown. Transfer into the slow cooker.
3. Add the remaining oil to the skillet. When the oil is heated, add onions and sauté until the onions are translucent.
4. Add garlic and oregano and sauté until fragrant. Add tomatoes and sauté for a while, mashing it simultaneously. Remove from heat.
5. Apply half this mixture over the lamb. Place the lamb in the slow cooker.
6. Place sweet potato slices over the lamb. Sprinkle salt and pepper. Next layer with green beans followed by eggplant. Place zucchini slices. Sprinkle salt and pepper over each layer.
7. Spread the remaining tomato mixture over the zucchini layer. Place the bay leaves.
8. Close the lid. Set cooker on 'Low' option and timer for 8-9 hours or on 'High' option and timer for 4-4 ½ hours.
9. Discard the bay leaves.
10. Ladle into bowls.
11. Garnish with parsley and serve.

Slow Cook Seafood Stew

Serves: 4

Preparation time: 20 minutes

Nutritional values per serving:

Calories - 215, Fat – 4 g, Carbohydrates – 15 g, Protein – 30 g

Ingredients:

- 3 ½ ounces canned clams, chopped, with its juices
- ½ pound shrimp, peeled, deveined
- 3 ounces canned crab meat, drained
- ½ pound firm white fish, cut into 1-inch pieces
- ½ tablespoon vegetable oil
- 1 medium stalk celery, chopped

- I large onion, chopped (about I cup)
- 14 ounces canned crushed tomatoes, with its liquid
- 3 cloves garlic, minced
- 4 ounces bottled clam juice
- ½ tablespoon red wine vinegar
- 3 ounces tomato paste
- ¼ cup dry white wine or water
- I bay leaf
- I ½ teaspoons dried basil
- I ½ teaspoons dried thyme
- I ½ teaspoons dried cilantro
- ¼ teaspoon red pepper flakes
- ¼ teaspoon cayenne pepper
- A handful fresh parsley, chopped

Method:

1. Add all the ingredients except seafood to the slow cooker. Mix well.
2. Close the lid. Set cooker on 'Low' option and timer for 6 hours or on 'High' option and timer for 3 hours.
3. Add the seafood and stir.
4. Cover and cook on 'High' for 30 minutes. Stir in between a couple of times while it is cooking. Taste and adjust the seasonings if necessary.

Keto Curried Carrot Soup

Serves: 3

Preparation time: 10 minutes

Nutritional values per serving:

Calories - 122, Fat – 7 g, Carbohydrates – 12 g, Protein – 4 g

Ingredients:

- I ½ tablespoons canola oil
- 4 medium carrots, peeled, thinly sliced

- 1 small onion, chopped
- 2 teaspoons lemon juice
- Freshly ground pepper to taste
- Salt to taste
- 1 teaspoon curry powder
- 2 medium stalks celery, thinly sliced
- 2 ½ cup low sodium vegetable or chicken broth

Method:

1. Place a skillet over medium heat. Add oil. When the oil is heated, add onions and sauté until translucent.
2. Add curry powder and sauté for a few seconds until fragrant.
3. Transfer into the slow cooker. Add the rest of the ingredients except lemon juice and stir.
4. Close the lid. Set cooker on 'Low' option and timer for 3-4 hours or on 'High' option and timer for 2 hours.
5. Blend with an immersion blender until smooth. Add lemon juice and stir.
6. Ladle into soup bowls and serve.

Real Mexican Chicken Soup

Serves: 3

Preparation time: 5 minutes

Nutritional values per serving:

Calories - 400, Fat – 22.8 g, Carbohydrates – 7.4 g, Protein – 38 g

Ingredients:

- ¾ pound chicken pieces, skinless, boneless
- 8 ounces chicken broth
- 8 ounces chunky salsa
- 4 ounces Monterey or Pepper Jack cheese, shredded

Method:

1. Add all the ingredients into the slow cooker and stir.

2. Close the lid. Set cooker on 'Low' option and timer for 3-4 hours or on 'High' option and timer for 2 hours.

3. Remove the chicken with a slotted spoon and place on your work area.

4. When cool enough to handle, shred with a pair of forks. Add chicken back into the pot.

5. Heat thoroughly. Ladle into soup bowls and serve.

Healthy Keto Chicken Stew

Serves: 6

Nutritional values per serving:

Calories - 228, Fat – 11 g, Carbohydrates – 6 g, Protein – 23 g

Ingredients:

- 14 ounces chicken, skinless, boneless, chopped into chunks
- 1 stick celery, chopped
- 2 small carrots, peeled, chopped into small pieces
- 1 cup mushrooms, quartered
- ¼ cup onion, chopped
- ¼ teaspoon dried rosemary
- ¼ teaspoon dried oregano
- ¼ teaspoon dried thyme
- 1 cup chicken stock
- ½ cup fresh spinach, chopped
- Salt and pepper to taste
- ¼ cup heavy cream
- 1/8 teaspoon xanthan gum or more
- 2 cloves garlic, minced

Method:

1. Add carrot, celery, chicken, garlic, herbs, stock into the slow cooker and stir.

2. Close the lid. Set cooker on 'Low' option and timer for 3-4 hours or on 'High' option and timer for 2 hours.

3. Add spinach, salt, pepper, and spinach.

4. Sprinkle some xanthan gum to get the desired thickness. Whisk well.

5. Heat thoroughly. Ladle into bowls and serve.

Mexican Green Chili Pork Stew

Serves: 4

Preparation time: 10 minutes

Nutritional values per serving:

Calories - 182, Fat – 10 g, Carbohydrates – 1 g, Protein – 20 g

Ingredients:

- 1 pound pork loin, cubed
- 1 teaspoon granulated garlic
- ¼ cup onion, chopped
- 13.5 ounces canned whole Hatch green chilies with its liquid
- 1 cup water
- 1 teaspoon ground cumin
- ½ teaspoon chili powder
- 1 clove garlic, sliced
- 4 teaspoons oil
- Salt to taste
- Fried or poached eggs (optional)

Method:

1. Place a skillet over medium heat. Add oil. When the oil is heated, add pork and sauté until brown. Remove with a slotted spoon and transfer to the slow cooker.

2. Add onions, garlic, and the chilies with its liquid into a blender. Blend until smooth. Pour over the pork in the slow cooker.

3. Add water and stir.

4. Close the lid. Set cooker on 'Low' option and timer for 7-8 hours or on 'High' option and timer for 3-4 hours.

5. Add cumin, chili powder, granulated garlic, and salt now. Stir well.

6. Ladle into bowls and serve with fried or poached eggs. (Nutritional value of egg is not included)

Turmeric Vegetable Beef Stew

Serves: 4-5

Preparation time: minutes

Nutritional values per serving:

Calories - 533, Fat – 39.5 g, Carbohydrates – 12.7 g, Protein – 31.9 g

Ingredients:

- 1 ¼ pounds beef braising, boneless, pat dried
- ½ cup vegetable broth or water
- 2 cloves garlic, peeled
- 1.1 pounds zucchini or marrow squash, diced
- ½ teaspoon ground ginger
- 1 tablespoon ground cumin
- ½ teaspoon ground coriander
- ½ tablespoon paprika
- ½ teaspoon chili powder
- ½ teaspoon turmeric powder
- 2 small onions, chopped
- 1 bay leaf
- Salt and freshly ground pepper to taste
- 1 teaspoon dried rosemary, crushed
- 1 stick cinnamon
- ¼ cup ghee or lard or tallow
- 7 ounces canned chopped tomatoes
- A handful parsley, chopped to garnish

Method:

1. Set the slow cooker on 'High' and preheat.
2. Sprinkle salt and pepper on the steaks.

3. Place a skillet over medium heat. Add a little ghee. Add 2 steaks and sauté until brown. Cook in batches. Remove with a slotted spoon and transfer to the slow cooker.

4. Add more ghee if required. Add onion and garlic and sauté until light brown. Add rest of the ingredients except zucchini and rutabaga and stir for a couple of minutes.

5. Transfer into the slow cooker. Stir well.

6. Close the lid. Set cooker on 'High' option and timer for 2 ½ hours.

7. Move the meat to one side of the slow cooker. Add rutabaga to the other side. Cover and cook for an hour. Discard bay leaf and cinnamon stick.

8. Place zucchini along with the rutabaga. Mix it lightly with the cooking liquid but do not mix the meat part. Cook for 1 ½ hours or until the vegetables are tender.

9. Serve in bowls. Garnish with parsley and serve.

Creamy Chipotle Tomato Soup

Serves: 3

Preparation time: 10 minutes

Nutritional values per serving:

Calories - 133, Fat – 5 g, Carbohydrates – 18 g, Protein – 5 g

Ingredients:

- 1 teaspoon olive oil
- 1 carrot, diced
- 1 clove garlic, minced
- 2 stalks celery, diced
- 1 medium onion, diced
- 2 tablespoons chipotle peppers
- 2 cups vegetable broth
- ½ teaspoon oregano
- 14 ounces canned whole tomatoes with its juice
- ¼ teaspoon ground cumin
- ¼ teaspoon ground coriander
- 1 bay leaf
- 4 tablespoons low-fat cream cheese
- Salt to taste
- ¾ cup non -fat milk

Method:

1. Place a skillet over medium heat. Add oil. When the oil is heated, add celery, carrot, and onions. Sauté until slightly soft.
2. Add garlic and chipotle pepper and sauté until fragrant. Transfer into the slow cooker.
3. Add rest of the ingredients except milk and cream cheese and stir.
4. Close the lid. Set cooker on 'Low' option and timer for 3-4 hours or on 'High' option and timer for 2 hours.
5. Discard bay leaf.
6. Blend with an immersion blender until smooth.
7. Add cream cheese and milk and stir. Cover and cook for 30-40 minutes.
8. Ladle into soup bowls and serve.

Chicken Masala with Cauliflower

Serves: 3

Preparation time: 10 minutes

Nutritional values per serving:

Calories - 289, Fat – 9 g, Carbohydrates – 15 g, Protein – g

Ingredients:

- ½ pound chicken breast, skinless, boneless, chopped
- ½ pound chicken thighs, skinless, boneless, chopped
- 1 teaspoon olive oil
- 2 teaspoons garlic paste
- 1 tablespoon tomato paste
- 1 teaspoon chili powder
- 1 onion, chopped
- 1 ½ cups cauliflower florets
- 2 teaspoons ginger paste
- 1 teaspoon garam masala (Indian spice blend)
- 14 ounces canned fire roasted tomatoes
- Salt to taste
- Cayenne pepper to taste, optional

* ½ cup light coconut milk

Method:

1. Place a skillet over medium heat. Add oil. When the oil is heated, add onions and sauté until light brown.
2. Add ginger and garlic and sauté until fragrant. Add tomato paste, salt and spices. Sauté for a couple of minutes until fragrant.
3. Add diced tomatoes and chicken. Mix well.
4. Transfer into the slow cooker.
5. Close the lid. Set cooker on 'Low' option and timer for 7-8 hours or on 'High' option and timer for 3-4 hours.
6. Add coconut milk and cauliflower during the last 30 minutes of cooking.
7. Mix well and serve.

Slow Cooked Ginger Chicken

Serves: 3

Preparation time: 10 minutes

Nutritional values per serving:

Calories – 225, Fat – 5 g, Carbohydrates – 10 g, Protein – 32 g

Ingredients:

* ½ pound chicken thigh, boneless, skinless
* ½ pound chicken breast, boneless, skinless
* 2 tablespoons chicken broth
* 2 teaspoons soy sauce or tamari
* 1 tablespoon stevia (optional)
* 1 tablespoon hoisin sauce
* 1 tablespoon orange juice
* 1 tablespoon fresh ginger, peeled, minced
* 2 cloves garlic, minced
* 3 teaspoons sesame seeds
* Salt to taste

Method:

1. Place the chicken in the slow cooker. Mix together rest of the ingredients except sesame seeds in a bowl and pour over the chicken.
2. Close the lid. Set cooker on 'Low' option and timer for 3-4 hours or on 'High' option and timer for 1 ½ -2 hours.

3. Remove the chicken with a slotted spoon and place on your work area. When cool enough to handle, slice or shred the chicken. Add the chicken back into the pot.

4. Uncover and cook for a while until the sauce thickens.

5. Sprinkle sesame seeds over it and serve.

Easy Curry Chicken Meatballs

Serves: 3

Preparation time: 15 minutes

Nutritional values per serving: 4 meatballs

Calories – 284, Fat – 15 g, Carbohydrates – 3 g, Protein – 33 g

Ingredients:

- 1 pound 95% lean ground chicken
- 1 tablespoon fresh cilantro, chopped
- 2 green onions, chopped
- 1 tablespoon fresh ginger, minced, divided
- 2 cloves garlic, minced, divided
- 2 tablespoons Thai green curry paste, divided or more to taste
- 1 cup light coconut milk
- 1 jalapeño, sliced (optional)
- 2 tablespoons almond meal
- 1 tablespoon fresh basil, chopped
- Salt to taste
- Pepper to taste
- ½ cup chicken broth

Method:

1. Add chicken, green onion, almond meal, cilantro, basil, half the ginger, garlic and Thai curry paste, salt, and pepper into a bowl and mix well.

2. Divide the mixture into 12 equal portions and shape into balls.

3. Add rest of the ingredients into the slow cooker and mix well. Lower the balls into the slow cooker.

4. Close the lid. Set cooker on 'Low' option and timer for 3-4 hours or on 'High' option and timer for 1 ½ -2 hours.

Conclusion

I hope this book was able to help you to achieve not only your weight loss goals, but to have a more vibrant, healthier lifestyle beyond losing weight and looking great.

This book and its contents, I hope, have been able to give you a structured and actionable step by step plan to start the diet.

More importantly, it is my hope as well that the book has also given you the confidence booster and built up the commitment to stay on the diet. The benefits of ketosis awaits, and if health is wealth, you should be getting wealthy pretty soon!

Finally, if you enjoyed this book, then I'd like to ask you for a favor, would you be kind enough to leave a review for this book on Amazon? It'd be greatly appreciated!

Thank you and good luck!

Anna Lovette

www.ingramcontent.com/pod-product-compliance
Lightning Source LLC
Chambersburg PA
CBHW081720250726
48657CB00010B/3066